what's
wrong
with the
mental health movement

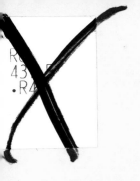
what's wrong with the mental health movement

K. Edward Renner, Ph.D.

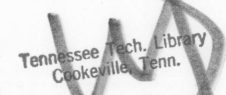

Nelson-Hall Publishers Chicago

Library of Congress Cataloging in Publication Data

Renner, K   Edward, 1936-
    What's wrong with the mental health movement

    (Professional/technical series)
    Includes indexes.
    1. Psychiatry—Philosophy. 2. Psychiatry—
Methodology. I. Title. [DNLM: 1. Mental Health.
2. Psychiatry. WM100 R414w]
RC437.5.R46   616.8'9'001   74-26831
ISBN 0-88229-180-7

Manufactured in the United States of America

table of contents

preface

This book is about the mental health movement. It is a highly personal account, based largely on my own experience and reflections.

The conceptual origins of the book go back some twelve years when I first began to treat psychiatric patients. The most significant impact on my early clinical work was the development of an acute awareness of certain contradictions within the mental health field.

In a psychiatric setting, many decisions are made each day about patients. Some of these decisions are relatively inconsequential. Others, however, have very important consequences for a particular individual—such decisions as whether or not to discharge; to attempt to give individual therapy or essentially to ignore the patient because of lack of staff; to give electro-convulsive shock treatment; or to commit the individual to a state hospital for long-term custodial care.

But, what was most remarkable to me was the air of certainty and infallibility with which these decisions were made. If the experience of going through a Ph.D. program in psychology had taught me anything, it was to evaluate the degree of certainty of what we know. And if anything was clear in the day-to-day operation of a clinical setting, it was the extensive and unquestioning reliance on concepts that were highly uncertain and fallible.

Of course, in an intellectual way, I knew that there was always a gap between knowledge in the pure sense and its application. Because the patients were there, someone had to decide, simply out of practical necessity. But why the air of certainty?

Clinical experience added a new dimension to my intellectual understanding. And, finally, the air of certainty began to make sense. It is very important to know that you are right when, as a therapist, you frequently make crucial decisions about other human beings. Certainty offers peace of mind to the clinician.

But there are other consequences that contradict the very purpose and goals the mental health field is supposed to serve. It is in this sense that the mental health worker becomes a malevolent benefactor. The sense of certainty that allows him to act, also creates conditions that are potentially dangerous and contrary to human well-being.

The contradiction can be seen in a number of ways. For example, a young, highly verbal, and educated patient is likely to be given individual attention, but a poor patient is often given electric-shock treatment or left largely on his or her own. There are elaborate concepts of personality, which when exercised with certainty, invariably show the first patient to have the potential for recovery. This seems to justify the allocation of limited human resources. Often the educated patient goes on to purchase further service as an outpatient.

But this kind of seemingly biased decision is not just one of economic self-interest. The mental health worker, who is also verbal and educated, is better able to relate to the first rather than to the poor patient. And, given our social reality, the chosen patient does have greater potential.

But these contradictions are not unique to the mental health profession. The same privilege is exercised where some individuals are given the opportunity to attend graduate, law, or medical school. These kinds of social injustices are not new, and although they are never to be condoned, it is hardly surprising to find that this discrimination exists in the mental health field. Certainty excludes the necessity of recognizing that the potential for recovery is as much a matter of economics as it is the infallibility of the knowledge.

Beyond this level of social justice, other contradictions are unique to the mental health field. At one level the professional sense of certainty has resulted in an overambitious extension and definition of the field. It has resulted in a willingness on the part of mental health practitioners to define an increasingly wider range of human events within their jurisdiction. Many social problems currently labeled as mental health problems could be viewed as other types of problems, problems that should be attended to by persons outside the mental health field. To define social problems as mental health problems is to hinder their solution; the label thus contradicts the stated aims and purposes of the mental health field.

And finally, the sense of certainty employed by the professionals has served to undermine the advancement of scientific knowledge upon which mental health service is presumably based. The very process of delivering and expanding the marketplace for mental health services has established an apparatus with its own momentum which contradicts the necessary inquiry to justify the expanded definition and associated services.

These contradictions are especially peculiar to the mental health field. What is more, they represent dangers not only to the individual consumer but to the public at large. If these contradictions are to be resolved in a constructive manner, it is necessary for the public to be more aware of their nature and rationale. It is toward this end that this book is dedicated.

My own solution was to move into pure research concerned with personality in general. From such a perspective, it is quite easy to surrender one's sense of certainty—for clinical decisions are especially remote to one engaged in research. There are no patients to deal with, no pressing day-to-day decisions, and no responsibility for the fate of other people. This distance can be an asset if it's used for detached critical analysis. It can also be a liability if it results in distortions of important realities of the practical situations or motivations of the people involved. I would hope that my previous experience as a clinician is vivid enough to avoid such distortions.

But the balance between critical analysis and empathy for individuals is delicate. And, although this book is critical of the mental health field, it is not my purpose to present mental health workers as having willfully evil intentions. Indeed, they are largely dedicated benefactors. But, by virtue of practical considerations and the history of the field, they also contribute to malevolent contradictions. These contradictions, in part, arise out of personal and practical dilemmas which need to be understood in their own right. Personal and practical considerations which give rise to the sense of certainty are given credence but not as an excuse or personal criticism of the people involved.

The book is an attempt to put the mental health field into perspective. I feel that the issues presented in this book belong in the public domain. They should not be confined to academic circles or to the practitioners. Only by including the general public in this discussion can the mental health field begin to be restructured. It is this writer's hope that the mental health expert can surrender his sense of certainty. In so doing, the mental health professional will open new areas of interaction with society. These experiences can help to alter the malevolent aspects of the supposedly benevolent mental health field.

Although the origins of the book began with my early clinical work, the actual manuscript was written while I was on sabbatical leave from the University of Illinois at the University of Waterloo, Ontario, Canada. I owe a special thanks to the faculty, students, and staff of Waterloo for providing a stimulating intellectual and warm social climate in which it was a delight to work and to exchange ideas.

1

introduction

Every subject has a history. But it is largely a matter of individual judgment in deciding where to begin an account of a subject so as to place it in the proper perspective. This arbitrary choice depends on the writer's views and his interpretation of past events. The selection of a starting point is important, however, because different vantage points are possible, and depending on the one selected, the areas of abnormal psychology may take rather different appearances.

I have just said that all things are relative. Everyone knows that. But because knowledge of the mental health field is changing rapidly, it is especially important to have a perspective, one that will determine how relevant a current fact is, was, or will be. Obtaining such a perspective requires a critical look at our beliefs. The evaluation must capture the context of the past and the issues of the future. It requires a focus on questions which have no absolute answers, and provide only a context with which to qualify our present knowledge and facts.

The psychology of abnormal behavior is at that stage of development where the issue of perspective is of paramount concern. There are several viewpoints, each distinct from the others. The most basic goal a student of abnormal behavior can aspire to is a healthy perspective, gained only by an objective inquiry into this temporary and ever-changing collection of facts and knowledge. This book presents a general perspective of the mental health field, contrary to the popular accepted view.

A starting point

The fifteenth century is a convenient beginning. One aspect of the late Middle Ages—witchcraft—is selected as the most relevant historical event. During the Middle Ages, madness was regarded as the work of the devil. Early Christian churches persecuted many innocent persons thought to be witches. The treatment was left to the priest, who attempted to relieve the sinner (mad person) by casting away the devil which possessed that person.

This religious campaign eventually took on frightful dimensions. Victims were tortured brutally. It has been estimated that some 300,000 women were put to death by the church in Europe between 1484-1782. Many confessed to being witches to avoid further abuse.

The elaborate procedures for the accusation and conviction of persons who allegedly had made a contract with the devil remain a dark period in human history. Many people who today are considered mentally ill, maladjusted, or at least strange or odd by the community were like those then accused of witchcraft.

2

In 1484, James Sprenger and Henry Kramer were appointed Inquisitors for all of Germany by Pope Innocent VIII, and in 1487 their manuscript entitled *Malleus Maleficarum* was officially approved by all the doctors of the theological faculty of the University of Cologne. [1] The purpose of Sprenger and Kramer's work was to define the nature and extent of behaviors that could result from forming a pact with the devil, and to describe the procedure to be used in dealing with such people. The book further established the proof that those so described were in fact in league with Satan. The book is replete with many examples of behaviors that today could easily be substituted for case histories illustrating various commonly recognized forms of psychopathology.

In describing the kinds of behavior that reflected the work of the devil, they wrote:

> And, finally . . . since the devil has power over inferior things, except only the soul, therefore he is able to effect certain changes in those things, when God allows, so that things appear to be otherwise than they are. And this he does, as I have said, either by confusing and deluding the organ of sight so that a clear thing appears cloudy. . . . Or by operating mental images, . . . Or by some agitation of various humors, so that matters which are earthy and dry seem to be fire or water. . . .

In addition, it was believed that witches had special powers to cause much evil. They were responsible for damage done by storms and other natural disasters. They were frequently accused of casting spells on other people, causing them personal misfortune or physical disability. Many of those who had spells cast on them would today be regarded as suffering from a hysterical or conversion reaction. As an example:

> . . . There was . . . an honest priest, who fondly held the opinion, or rather error, that there was no witchcraft

in the world . . . And God wished so to purge him of this error that he might even be made aware of the practice of devils in setting a term to the lives of witches. For as he was hastening to cross a bridge . . . he met a certain old woman in his hurry, and would not give way to her, but pressed on so that he thrust the old woman into the mud. She indignantly broke into a flood of abuse, and said to him, "Father, you will not cross with impunity." And though he took small notice of those words, in the night, when he wished to get out of his bed, he felt himself bewitched below the waist, so that he always had to be supported by the arms of other men . . . and so he remained for three years, under the care of his own mother. After that time the old woman fell sick, . . . and it happened that she sent to him to hear her confession . . . And . . . two servants listened outside the window, so eager were they to know whether she would confess that she had bewitched the priest . . . she said "Father, do you know who bewitched you?" . . . she added, "you suspect me, and with reason; for know that I brought it upon you for this reason," explaining as we have already told. And when he begged to be liberated, she said, "Lo! the set time has come and I must die; but I will so cause it that in a few days, after my death, you will be healed." . . . For she died at the time fixed by the devil, and within thirty days the priest found himself completely healed . . . .

And, regarding sexual incapacity, now commonly regarded as a psychosomatic disorder:

. . . Nider tells of a wizard . . . who . . . confessed that in a certain house where a man and his wife were living, he had by his witchcraft successively killed in the woman's womb seven children, so that for many years the woman always miscarried . . . . And when he was questioned as to how he had done this, and what manner of charge should be preferred against him, he discovered his crime, saying: I put a serpent under the threshold of the outer door of the house; and if this is removed, fecundity will be restored to the inhabitants. And it was as he said; for though the serpent was not found, having been reduced to dust, the whole piece of ground was removed, and in the same year fecundity was restored . . . .

And finally, it should be noted that these facts and knowledge were not a form of madness itself, but a carefully and thoughtfully arrived at "truth." The position was well supported by a host of indisputable facts:

> But . . . on the next day the other witch had at first been exposed to the very gentlest questions, being suspended hardly clear off the ground by her thumbs, after she had been set quite free, she disclosed the whole matter . . . . .

And in another instance:

> . . . suddenly, when she had been freed from her chains, although it was in the torture chamber, she fully laid bare all the crimes which she had committed.

The author concluded that:

> These instances must serve, since indeed countless examples of this sort of mischief could be recounted. But very often men and beasts and storehouses are struck by lightning by the power of devils . . . . However, it has been found that witches have freely confessed that they have done such things . . . .

The legal system for conviction for witchcraft (the parallel today is involuntary hospitalization) was such that a witch could be given the death penalty on the basis of (1) confession; (2) testimony of respected others; or (3) evidence that proved the guilt. However, confession was regarded as good for the witch, because it put her on better terms with God. Thus confession—apart from its validating value—was also a treatment. Accordingly, if a death penalty were involved, the judge could first sentence her to be questioned and tortured, and could even promise the accused her life if she confessed, although the promise was often false and used only to obtain the confession. The instructions for con-

ducting this determination of witchcraft were given
in some detail:

> . . . Let him summon her friends and put it to them
> that she may escape the death penalty, although she will
> be punished in another way, if she confesses the truth,
> and urge them to try and to persuade her to do so. For
> very often meditation, and the misery of imprisonment,
> and the repeated advice of honest men, dispose the
> accused to discover the truth . . .
>
> But if, after keeping the accused in a state of
> suspense, and continually postponing the day of
> examination, and frequently using verbal persuasions, the
> Judge should truly believe that the accused is denying the
> truth, let them question her lightly . . . .
>
> And it should be begun in this way. While the officers
> are preparing for questioning, let the accused be strip-
> ped . . . they should search for any instrument of
> witchcraft sewn into her clothes . . . . And . . . the Judge
> shall use his own persuasion . . . to induce her to confess
> the truth voluntarily; and if she will not, let him order the
> officers to bind her with cords, and apply her to some
> engine of torture . . . . Then let her be released again at
> someone's earnest request, and taken on one side, and let
> her again be persuaded; and in persuading her, let her be
> told that she can escape the death penalty.
>
> Here it is asked whether, in the case of a prisoner
> legally convicted by her general bad reputation, by
> witnesses, and by the evidence of the fact, so that the only
> thing lacking is a confession of the crime from her own
> mouth, the Judge can lawfully promise her life, whereas if
> she were to confess the crime she would suffer the
> extreme penalty.
>
> . . . some hold that if the accused is of a notoriously
> bad reputation, and gravely suspected on unequivocal
> evidence of the crime; and if she is herself a great source
> of danger, as being the mistress of other witches, then she
> may be promised her life on the following conditions: that
> she be sentenced to imprisonment for life on bread and
> water, provided that she supply evidence that will lead to
> the conviction of other witches. And she is not to be told,
> when she is promised her life, that she is to be imprisoned
> in this way; but should be led to suppose that some other

> penance, such as exile, will be imposed on her as punishment . . . .
>
> Others think that, after she has been consigned to prison in this way, the promise to spare her life should be kept for a time, but after a certain period she should be burned . . . .
>
> But if neither threats nor such promises will induce her to confess the truth, then . . . .
>
> The next step of the Judge should be that, if after being fittingly tortured she refuses to confess the truth, he should have other engines of torture brought before her, and tell her that she will have to endure these if she does not confess. If then she is not induced by terror to confess, the torture must be continued . . . .

This procedure had the misguided effect of discovering new witches, of treating the souls of those already convicted, and providing further evidence of the relationship between madness and a pact with the devil. It falsely confirmed the danger witches presented to society and provided a further justification for the procedure. As was apparent for those involved, there was a theoretical account of madness which they accepted as based on factual information and a form of treatment and disposition which followed from theory. Yet, how unjust and cruel and evil were those clergymen who could accuse, torture, and kill persons allegedly in concert with the devil. Significantly, it was all accomplished with legality and certainty.

The first American institution to treat the mentally ill was Pennsylvania Hospital, founded in 1751. As the problem of devils moved from the church's sphere of influence to a problem of illness in the domain of medicine, there was a strong carryover in the actual applied approach. For example, Dr. Benjamin Rush, the director of Pennsylvania Hospital, and sometimes called the father of American psychiatry, noted that "...terror acts powerfully on the body through the medium of the mind, and should be employed in the cure of madness." [2] The treatment of disease by the administration of punishment has a long history in medicine. It was based on the assumption that disease represented a punishment for sin and could be relieved only through atonement. The tradition extended to the early treatment of mental illness in which near drowning, rapid and repeated swinging of a person in a circle and other such treatments were used as a means for driving from the mind whatever ailed it.

It's not difficult to see an underlying theoretical orientation that made such practices seem reasonable. Medical history is full of similar treatments for madness which once were considered humanitarian and helpful.

The point to be underscored is this: *what we do depends heavily on what we think we know.* This is no less true now than before. It is a simple matter of translating theory into action. The instant we isolate a group of people and call them witches (mad, mentally ill, or what have you), we do so only by making numerous assumptions and judgments. Once we start to do something to people to change them, we make even more assumptions about the basis of the behavior we seek to change. A theoretical view of some kind is implicit in current concepts of mental illness just as one was implicit in the past approach to witchcraft. We need to be as explicit as possible about our assumptions if we are to learn efficiently from our experience.

Modern psychiatry

This morbid story of witches is in the past. Unfortunately, modern concepts of madness have not kept pace with the growth in sophistication of man's knowledge in general. Physical treatments have remained popular until the last decade or two; since then they have been increasingly replaced by the use

8

of drugs, known as chemical therapy. The slow progression from 1484 to the 1940s and 1950s can be illustrated by describing several of the more recent and widely used forms of physical treatment.[3]

One such form of physical treatment was electro-convulsive shock therapy, developed in 1938 for use in the treatment of schizophrenics. The apparatus permits the doctor to select a voltage of shock, usually between 70 to 130 volts, to be administered for a specified duration, usually from .1 to .5 of a second. A new patient may be started at 80 volts for .2 of a second. The voltage may be adjusted upward on subsequent applications to achieve a generalized seizure.

The shock is administered while the patient is lying on his back with his arms and legs held in place to prevent extreme movements at the time of shock. The limbs must not be held too rigidly because a bone fracture could result; a padded tongue depressor is used to prevent biting the tongue. The gag must be held in place and the chin held firmly to prevent the jaw from becoming dislocated.

The electric shock is administered between electrodes placed on the temples of the patient. After this treatment, there is an impairment of the patient's memory. The memory loss may vary from a mild tendency to forget things, to severe confusion, depending on the number of days the patient has received shock treatments. The loss tends to cover a long time prior to treatment but gradually diminishes to the events just before treatment. The memory loss may continue for weeks or even months following treatment, although full return of memory does occur. Electric shock treatment does not alter intellectual performance.

Another physical treatment, known as psychosurgery or lobotomy, consists of surgically severing the connection between the thalamus and the frontal lobe. In 1936 the lobotomy procedure was first introduced, and in 1949, the developer of the procedure received the Nobel Prize in medicine for his work. The surgery severs the fibers, reducing the emotional component of the mental disturbance so it no longer dominates behavior, but leaves a sufficient quantity of the frontal lobes to permit a capacity for productive work. This operation obviously alters intellectual capacity.

After the operation, there is often an exaggeration of some unpleasant traits. Friends and relatives must be prepared to overlook the patient's sarcastic remarks and undesirable behavior. The patient will not be self-conscious or facetious and is often likely to show a childlike pleasure in simple things. The patient should probably not ever assume financial responsibility or attempt unusual social adjustments. At best the patient loses his anxiety, becomes friendly, takes an interest in himself, and may work regularly but without ambition. At worst, there is no improvement in the clinical condition and a permanent loss of intelligence.

A prefrontal lobotomy is a radical procedure and its use as a treatment has greatly decreased since the introduction of tranquilizing drugs. However, because of recent discoveries of techniques for exploring the brain, there has been a resurgence of interest in psychosurgery, but now directed at small specific parts of the brain. In fact, in 1970 an international conference on psychosurgery was attended by some one hundred psychosurgeons to discuss recent developments in the field.

These developments now include procedures for recording brain patterns from wires implanted in the brain of fully conscious patients, for stimulating areas found to have abnormal patterns to see if they are associated with verbal reports of troublesome thoughts or emotions, and for electrically destroying those small areas identified as possible sources of the problem. Because the procedure requires probing the interior of the brain with small wires, it may take four to six hours for an operation and several such sessions may be needed. A vital aspect of this new procedure is the exchange of research information and case studies which suggest which parts of the brain, what pattern of recordings, and which amounts and kinds of destruction of brain tissue are associated with particular forms of behavior and emotions. Of particular interest has been violence and rage in adults and constant and impulsive activity in children. This technique, and others to be presented later, are being considered as ways to treat criminals before they commit acts of violence and to help children before they are school failures.

Commentary

Electro-convulsive therapy is still used, although less frequently than during the 1940s and 1950s. One reason for this decline is the development of tranquilizing drugs. It is now possible to control patients and relieve anxiety without the unwanted side effects, such as loss of orientation and memory with shock, or loss of motivation with surgery. Thus, the physical therapies were replaced by chemical therapies which achieve similar effects more easily. Drugs are likely to be tried first and shock treatment used only when the response to the drugs is insufficient. However, this pattern appears to be changing. Increasingly, treatments now are intended to deal with social problems rather than personal anxiety and traditional mental symptoms. And, recent advances in brain research have given rise to new forms of psychosurgery directed at specific areas of the brain. In hearings held before the Senate Committee on Labor and Public Welfare on February 23, 1973, the director of the National Institute of Mental Health estimated that as many as 1000 psychosurgery operations are performed yearly in the United States, and other testimony indicated that the number is increasing.

A parallel was intended between the concepts and practices used for treating witches and the relatively recent practice of prefrontal surgery; the still used practice of electric shock; and the new psychosurgery. The increased sophistication represented by the change from the treatments of the Inquisition to the recent physical therapies is not as great as the change from bows and arrows to the level of understanding represented by the space age.

Today, more people leave psychiatric hospitals and resume their previous lifestyle sooner than was ever true before. The final percentage of patients who remain well, however, may not be much better than it ever was because many who are discharged have to return. But at least, according to our current beliefs about madness, the treatment is more humane. Patients are not subjected to abuse and the treatment apparently does not cause pain.

In the future, however, current physical therapies may seem primitive because they are not based on a clear knowledge of the behavioral phenomenon, whether it's called witchcraft or mental illness. Most of our therapeutic advances are primarily technological advances. We have found ways to move people out of the hospitals faster, but we have not made a great deal of conceptual advancement.

For example, we do not understand just what effect electro-convulsive shock therapy has on the brain; we do not know from either a neurological or psychological point of view why such treatment techniques seem to work in some cases. There is not a great deal of difference between an effect described in 1489 as one which ". . .operates on the imaginative faculty by a transmutation of mental images. . ." and one describing electric shock in 1963 as one altering ". . .affective responses [so] that

tensions do not accumulate. . . ." In a sense, we
have cast out the mental illness in much the same
respect as early priests cast out the demons, i.e., the
madness.

At some future time, the physical therapies are
likely to seem punitive. In one of the wards in the
hospital where I served my psychology internship in
1960, nearly every patient received electro-
convulsive shock therapy. The motto of the unit, *à la*
Westinghouse, was "live better electrically." The
procedure of administering the treatment was so
perfected that fifteen patients could receive their
shocks in what I imagine was the period that in old
times was required to elevate a single person off the
ground by the thumbs. Such a comparison is unfair
perhaps, because the electro-convulsive shocks were
administered by well-meaning physicians concerned
about the mental health of the patient. But, the
witchcraft trials were likewise administered by
agents of the church, concerned about the soul and
its immortal existence.

The problems and issues that today face the
mental health researcher, the theoretician, and the
practitioner have relevance in a historical comparison. There are many such problems and issues. But they center principally on an evaluation
of our current knowledge and practices for dealing
with mental illness. The rest of this book is devoted
to the elaborations and the qualifications that are
necessary to put this historical comparison into a
perspective so that one may gain from the vantage
point.

The task is to explore the level of sophistication
that has been achieved to date, for it is on these
grounds that we must make our decisions. These
decisions include how first to conceptualize and then
treat madness, how to allocate resources by
choosing between various alternatives, and what
social values have a bearing on the problem. Only

with such a perspective is it possible to understand the directions that current psychological and psychiatric research and practice are taking, and to come to grips more precisely with the basic issues and problems. I hope to bring some of these unresolved issues and problems more sharply into focus.

2

a
brief
historical
perspective

The first chapter suggested the similarity between the past and the present in terms of the sophistication of our concepts and values concerning mental health. There have been changes, however, both in the content of our concepts and in the actions which seem to follow. The similarity between witches and mental illness can be shown by tracing the historical origin of ideas about mental illness. A brief perspective will be presented in terms of three contexts. The purpose is to illustrate some of the reasons why progress in dealing with mental illness has been so slow and why the comparison with concepts of 1487 is reasonable.

Historical trends

The idea that abnormal behavior was the result of an organic disease was the dominant line of thinking during the early 1900s. This view was expressed in the writings of Emil Kraeplin (1855-1926) who was the most influential psychiatrist of the period.[1] The disease concept of mental illness received its support from the discovery that a prevalent form of a progressively deteriorating mental disorder, known as general paresis, was caused by a syphilitic infection of the central nervous system. The basic relationship was established at the turn of the century. In 1906, August von Wassermann, a German bacteriologist, developed a test which showed that syphilitic antibodies were present in the cerebral-spinal fluid of general paretics. By 1913, the syphilitic organism was located in the brain tissue.[2] The discovery that a particular form of abnormal behavior had a specific cause had a strong influence on scientific thought because it was believed that similar kinds of causes could be found for all other forms of mental illness. Madness, consequently, was to be seen as a by-product of infection.

Investigators tried to find a similar basis for the other mental disorders. Kraeplin was committed to a belief that underlying each mental disorder was an organic agent. He tried to group illnesses into categories on the basis of their symptoms because he thought that in this way he could identify common groups of patients with a common cause. Kraeplin carefully observed large numbers of psychiatric patients. On the basis of their behavior, he concluded that there were two major types of mental disorders—Manic-depressive psychosis and schizophrenia. However, his hope of finding a common physical cause was never realized.

Fundamental to any classification effort is the

assumption that by categorizing patients on the basis of their disturbed behavior, one might be able to discover the basic etiological agent. The hypothesis of an organic basis of disturbed behavior was the dominant view in the early 1900s. It is to Kraeplin's credit that his careful observation of patients provided the basis for a categorization that is still used today. Note that his is a *descriptive* system only. It describes the patient's behavior in terms of symptoms that seem to go together. The implications of descriptive diagnostic systems will be considered in depth in Chapter Five. For now, it is sufficient to note that patients are assumed to be similar, not on the basis of underlying causes, but because of some symptomatic behavior that they share in common with other patients.

In contrast to the organic hypothesis is a psychological hypothesis. This alternative looks to the unique life experiences of the individual that produced the disturbed behavior. The view that the causes of abnormal behavior are psychological in origin can be traced to the early work of an Austrian physician, Franz Mesmer (1734-1815), in his studies of hypnosis. Mesmer, through hypnotic suggestion, showed that a subject can be made to have false sensations, such as hearing or seeing things that are not present, or experiencing anesthesia so as to feel no pain from a pinprick. Today, hypnosis is being used with growing frequency as an anesthetic in dentistry and for childbirth. Mesmer showed that many forms of mental illness, such as paralysis and physical complaints, could be changed through suggestion, which was a purely psychological technique. However, his theory was not psychological. He believed that the planets influenced the human body through a universal magnetic fluid, and the distribution of this fluid caused either health or disease. He felt that he was using his own magnetic fluid to influence others and effect cures.

However, his explanation was not taken seriously, even in his own time. The significance of Mesmer's findings was that apparently disabling symptoms, for example, paralysis of a leg or an arm, could be treated or cured through hypnosis. No physical treatment was given to the body itself but patients were relieved of their symptoms or suffering merely by hypnosis and the suggestion that the defect would no longer exist.

The work of Mesmer in the late 1700s provided the background for a psychological view of the origins of abnormal behavior. Hysteria is a form of disorder in which a physical symptom such as paralysis of an arm, blindness, or anesthesia may appear in some part of the body. As knowledge about the physiological make-up of the body increased, it became apparent to a few physicians that there was something unique about hysteria. For example, there was no atrophy of a limb that wasn't used, or if there was a paralysis or lack of sensation, it did not follow the nerve patterns of the body. In other words, the paralysis or dysfunction didn't make anatomical sense.

Later, Pierre Janet (1859-1947), a French neurologist, reported a case known as Irene. In her conscious state, the patient had forgotten the death of her mother, but occasionally would go into a dreamy state and act out the death scene. Janet introduced the concept of dissociation to explain this behavior. By this term he meant there was a breaking up of thoughts and memories into isolated parts or systems. Clearly, his idea of dissociation was only descriptive, for he simply labeled what he observed happening: that some parts of the personality system seemed to be isolated from others.

Implicit in Janet's work, however, was some indecision about choosing between a psychological or an organic explanation. He eventually leaned toward an explanation of aberrant behavior based on hereditary weakness; a personal failure to organize the different aspects of one's personality. But the concept of dissociation showed it was possible for a person to have a splitting or division of the personality into separate systems.

It remained for others, especially Sigmund Freud, to suggest that hysterical disorders had psychological rather than physiological origins. Based on his own experience, Freud developed an explanation of the psychological nature of hysteria. His basic discoveries were made in the late 1800s, although he did not work out the details of his theory until later. The basic ingredient of his psychological explanation of abnormal behavior and its attendant symptoms was strong emotion that had been suppressed. He believed that when the emotional event could be recovered and released by the patient, the symptom would be removed.

As an example, a woman who had strong emotional feelings of resentment toward her husband suppressed those feelings because they were in conflict with her religious and moral values. The conflict found expression in a phobia of anything sharp. Symbolically, the sharp instrument represented a means to express her hostility, but the fear of the instrument represented the need to deny that resentment. Eventually the woman became a patient with overt symptoms who found normal functioning impossible. Once the intense emotional feeling was recovered and brought into awareness, the symptom was relieved. Freud saw such symptoms only as a symbolic outlet for the psychological energy consumed by the underlying conflict.

In this case there was a basis for a dynamic view of pathological behavior, with the symptoms being the unconscious manifestations of unexpressed emotional energy. The removal of the symptom depended upon release of the emotion.

It was observations such as these on the role of

suppressed unconscious emotional forces which led Freud to develop his theory of psychopathology. His approach was radically different from the organic "illness" hypothesis previously considered. Freud placed the responsibility for abnormal behavior squarely upon the life experiences of the patient. He asserted that psychological factors could lead to such things as the dissociation of personality into isolated subsystems, and that psychological factors could influence the total functioning of the patient.

Frued's theory at this point was simple. Repressed emotional experiences produced abnormal symptoms through unconscious processes. The recovery and full expression of the emotion would free an individual of his or her symptoms. The basis for modern dynamic psychiatry was laid down in the early 1900s by Freud. Freud modified his system until his death, but by the 1920s his basic theory of human personality development was completed.

Initially there was great resistance to Freud's ideas. At the same time that Freud was presenting his ideas, the organic hypothesis achieved significant strength by the discovery of the connection between a syphilitic infection and general paresis. In any case, a psychological hypothesis was not appealing to the scientific community.

It took World War I to establish further the psychological basis of neurotic behavior. Under combat stress, some individuals developed symptoms which paralleled civilian abnormal behavior. By the end of World War I, at least some medical people saw that symptoms such as disorientation, physical complaints, and uncontrollable fear could be the result of psychological factors. The stress that combat troops were under was one good example. These observations provided the basis for some support within the scientific community for Freud's notions. Nevertheless, by 1920 there were few who were professionally concerned with psychiatry, and the field of clinical psychology did not exist. Mental hospitals did exist, but very little treatment, if any, was given. The hospitals were dominated by Kraeplin's concept that the disorders were due to organic factors that had not yet been discovered. Treatment could not be given since the nature of the infection was unknown.

It wasn't until approximately 1935 that Freud's insights gained a sufficient following to make their full impact felt, and thus only in the post-1935 era did the field of abnormal psychology begin to emerge. This, perhaps, marks the beginning of the time when patients were viewed as having a disturbance primarily in their psychological functions. When these functions could be opened to investigation and study, they could reflect the patient's past histories, including their experiences, rather than some form of infectious disease.

World War II provided another demonstration of the power of psychological factors in producing abnormal behavior. A psychological viewpoint was further established as a consequence of the war when the federal government supported the training of clinical psychologists to help provide professional manpower for the treatment of patients in Veteran's Administration hospitals.

This brief historical account illustrates how dynamic thinking has evolved. The point is simple. A view of abnormal behavior as a disturbance of psychological processes is relatively new. Freud made a major contribution by establishing a unique position about how man viewed himself. He achieved this against a hostile background, working alone much of the time. Very little of the basis for his discovery was provided by other investigators. The uniqueness of his position is perhaps best illustrated by the initially cold reception his ideas received from the scientific community. It took until approximately 1935 before there was a grudging acceptance of a psychological basis for abnormal behavior. Only then did important scientific work begin on the nature of psychological disturbances.

Two positions for viewing abnormal behavior have been outlined. The first focuses on a medical illness and carries the connotation of a disease. The second focuses on psychological factors and puts the emphasis on problems in living. Each position still has supporters. The illness viewpoint has never been completely supplanted and is gaining some support via the use of the physical therapies and the use of tranquilizing drugs in psychiatric hospitals today. Current ideas are more sophisticated than those involving general paresis, but the basic notion is that a dysfunctioning physiological, biochemical, or central nervous system is responsible. The psychological viewpoint is equally strong but has now divided into two camps. The traditional camp has extended the work and the type of concepts Freud proposed. It will be referred to as the *dynamic* position. The more recent position that provides the other psychological orientation will be referred to as the *behavioral* position.

The behavioral position is in agreement with the dynamic on the importance of psychological explanations but disagrees with the particular approach of Freud. Freud's concepts are rejected because it is believed that they do not provide an adequate theory of human personality. Much of this book is concerned with evaluating the differences between these two positions.

The discussion of historical trends in scientific circles shows that we have not progressed a great deal since the Middle Ages in our theoretical understanding of abnormal behavior. We are still in the position of establishing the general direction to pursue. It is difficult to know by what yardstick to judge progress.

Trends in public attitudes

Once assumptions are made about a certain phenomenon, other things will naturally follow. Scientific theories are assumptions about aspects of our experience. If one assumes a psychological point of view, mental disorders seem very different than they would if one accepted an illness point of view.

In the early 1800s, people we would now call mentally ill were treated as social outcasts. The very best that could be hoped for was to be regarded as of weak character or out of touch with God (and, therefore, being punished by God for wrong deeds). The patient lost his standing and the respect of his community; he or she was bad and should feel guilty about his or her symptoms.

Then, a few people began to see madness differently—as an illness. In a limited sense, there was some change in the public attitude toward the mentally ill—from sinner to patient status. This change was brought about in the United States primarily because of Dorothea Dix (1802-1887), a Quaker and a retired schoolteacher from Boston. She visited jails and poorhouses near Boston in the early 1840s and discovered that the harmlessly insane were confined in filthy pens and cages, chained, and beaten with rods. She was able to gain publicity for her cause by writing articles for newspapers exposing the horror she witnessed. She spent the last half of her life working to improve the tragic lot of the mentally ill. She visited state legislatures to plead her cause that the insane should be treated in public hospitals established and supported by the states, and not abandoned in foul local jails and poorhouses where the mentally ill were regarded as sinners, complete failures as human beings. This attitude toward the insane perhaps provided an explanation, if not justification, as to why and how

such inhuman physical punishment could be inflict-
ed. Dorothea Dix went before many other state
legislatures and was able to convince them that it
was the state's responsibility to provide hospital care
for the mentally deranged. Such liberalism was not
far-reaching, but it was obviously a clear step ahead
in concept, if not in practice. Because, in fact, the
new hospitals soon became overcrowded and many
of the old abuses were reinstated.

The mental health movement received its next
boost from a former mental patient by the name of
Clifford Beers who wroted a book entitled, *The Mind
That Came Back.* Beers campaigned during the
early 1900s for better mental health facilities. He
described the cruel ways in which patients were
treated and the filth and abuse they suffered. The
maltreatment was probably contributed to by the
fact that patients were cared for by workers who still
regarded them as people with moral weaknesses.
Beers finally raised the question of how *badly*
patients were treated in these hospitals, so that
finally mental patients were considered as fellow
human beings who deserved to be treated as such. It
was a radically new idea.

A coincidence of scientific progress had an
impact in the early 1900s. Within medical circles, the
organic assumption was on the upswing because of
the discovery of the role of syphilis in one form of
mental disorder. Presumably, all patients had an
infection like syphilis, but one which simply had not
been discovered yet. Given this state of knowledge,
there was nothing to do but wait. Accordingly,
mental hospitals were built in the country, far away
from the city, where fresh air and sunshine were in
abundance. The patients were expected to farm the
land and thereby help to pay their way much as
convicts in penal institutions did. A by-product of this
was the isolation of patients from major medical
centers where there was adequately trained manpower.

Hospitals became storage bins—literally and conceptually. Literally, because there were many more patients than space. Conceptually, because an organ that has been destroyed by infection is a hopeless cause. Mental patients were kept in out-of-the-way places, away from public concern and competent physicians. There was little money, no staff, and few new ideas.

The Snake Pit by Mary Jane Ward, published in 1946, and Albert Deutsch's *The Shame of the States* in 1948, brought to the public's attention the idea that mental patients were indeed people and entitled to decent treatment. Numerous other examples of responsible reporting came to the public's attention. In Deutsch's book, a photograph showing a ward of Byberry Hospital in Philadelphia was repulsive. [3]

The caption read:

> The male "incontinent ward" was like a scene out of Dante's *Inferno.* Three hundred nude men stood, squatted and sprawled in this bare room, amid shrieks, groans, and unearthly laughter. These represented the most deteriorated patients. Winter or summer, these creatures never were given any clothing at all. Some lay about on the bare floor in their own excreta. The filth-covered walls and floor were rotting away. Could a truly civilized community permit humans to be reduced to such animal-like level?

Deutsch reported that these dreadful conditions existed in a state that had a treasury surplus of $200 million, yet the pay for hospital attendants was $69 a month plus partial maintenance. The working conditions were hardly ideal. Today, we debate about what the public's responsibility should be in terms of welfare payments and prison reform.

Legislators have, over the years, been generally reluctant to provide funds for mental health facilities. Public attitudes have been slow to change. But since 1948, some improved facilities have been provided. With the passage of the Community Mental Health Act of 1963, a number of patients were moved to hospitals closer to their families and also nearby large medical complexes. Within the last several decades, there has been a noticeable effort to provide better facilities in some of the states.

But the question remains: Why has progress been so slow? There are probably many reasons, but the answer has to be assigned in part to the attitude of the general public—ashamed to admit the existence of mental illness and slow to accept the fact that such illness is a societal problem. Over the past ten years, there has been a quiet campaign to create a different public attitude. Television commercials announced, "Mental illness can happen to anyone—it can be treated." Also, "A troubled person needs a friend." But only now are we in the process of witnessing a transition in public attitudes toward the mentally ill from one of public charge to public responsibility. In terms of attitudes, mental illness has changed from something to be ashamed of to something that happens to people.

One way to measure the public concern is by the conditions in mental hospitals today. We would all, I am sure, like to think that the majority of our present facilities are modern and well-staffed. But, many are not. Life in many of the regressive wards of state hospitals is not much better than it was fifteen or twenty years ago—peeling paint, falling plaster, loose and missing floor tiles, little sunlight, hard oak chairs and benches—not to mention the many persons laying on the floor in their own excrement, and the prevailing smell of human urine that brings a wave of nausea to the occasional visitor. The image from these back wards is of human tragedy. My own visits always serve as a harsh reminder of how far removed from common decency are those foul-smelling wards.

Of course, by now, most states have a showplace hospital, typically a shiny new building located near an urban medical and research center that literally bustles with the enthusiastic efforts of a competent and efficient staff using new and imaginative treatment ideas. I worked in such a shiny hospital once. It held 250 patients distributed over a large space so that each patient could receive some individual attention. Nevertheless, the majority of mental patients are still confined in out-of-the-way storage bins left over from the early 1900s. At these hospitals, many wards have as many as 250 patients or more, and somewhere between ten to twenty such wards in one hospital. These hospitals have a generally incompetent staff, which in total size is almost certainly smaller than the showcase hospital has for 250 patients.

What kind of treatment and facilities are patients entitled to? How should public resources be allotted? As public attitudes change, so do the kinds of action that are taken toward mental illness. Mental health is not farther along today because the problem has not been presented to the public in such a way as to demand new solutions. In this sense, the distance between mental illness and witchcraft is relatively small.

There is still another way of looking at the problem. The statistics that follow will serve as a commentary on the current state of knowledge and describe the extent of mental illness and its treatment in the United States.

Dimensions and resources

In 1955, the U.S. Congress empowered the Joint Commission on Mental Illness and Health to conduct the first national study of our mental health resources and needs. The final report of this commission appeared in 1961.

Until that report, there had been no adequate

statistics available to document either the extent of the problem or the resources. It was in 1961, for the first time, that descriptive statistics could be used as the basis for decisions, actions, and allocation of resources. The facts revealed by this study were by no means encouraging.

At the time of that report, over one million people were hospitalized annually for psychiatric reasons; this figure did not include institutionalized mental defectives, epileptics, or the aged. The number increased from 153 per 100,000 of the population in 1961 to 175 per 100,000 in 1974. On any given day, there are about 746,000 hospitalized psychiatric patients in all the mental hospitals, public and private, in the United States. The difference between the yearly and daily total indicates that about 50,000 patients die each year in mental hospitals and other patients replace those who have been discharged. The replacements are new patients admitted for the first time as well as readmissions—persons who were previously discharged but who have had a relapse.

The relative size of the mental health problem can be best illustrated by some comparisons. One-half of all the hospital beds in the United States are occupied by psychiatric patients. These figures do not include those patients who are hospitalized for physical illnesses and complaints that may be entirely or partly due to psychological factors. The percentage of this type of patient in general medical hospital beds has been estimated to be anywhere from 25 to 50 percent of all hospital beds. These figures do not include psychiatric patients who do not require hospital beds but receive treatment on an outpatient basis or from someone in private practice.

The statistics indicated that most people pay little attention to mental health. Only after the 1961 report were efforts begun to rectify that situation; in particular the passage of the Community Mental

Health Act of 1963, which supported new staff and buildings.

Even so, mental health needs have had to compete with other public needs (including our continuing Southeast Asian involvement) for limited amounts of money. Since it takes about four to five years of graduate work to produce a Ph.D. psychologist, the rate of growth is further constrained. Progress cannot be pushed beyond some limit, even if the resources are available.

The simple fact is that there are many patients, few facilities, fewer personnel, and many professionals concentrated in large cities selling their services to individuals on a private, outpatient basis. Still not mentioned are the 17 million unhospitalized people the Commission has estimated to be suffering from some mental disorder. And nothing has been said about the suicides, or the welter of related problems—only about the hospitalized. The numbers speak for themselves. Until recently, what has been called the mental health field has been largely ignored.

Given this background, it is appropriate to summarize the recommendations of the Joint Commission. These recommendations were for greater support for the acquisition of basic knowledge of the field, better facilities for patients, and more resources to train qualified manpower.

Commentary

This chapter was not intended as a crusade for a massive social action program. No particular form of action is obvious, many are possible, including maintaining the status quo. Clearly, what is appropriate depends on a variety of values—social, ethical, economic, and political. What is appropriate also depends on information input from the biological and social sciences. The relevance of mental illness to our everyday life is, in part, a matter of definition involving beliefs and attitudes. The church chose to assume responsibility for those whom they accused of witchcraft. Now on secular grounds, psychiatric patients have come to be regarded as the responsibility of the state.

The decisions of the past were guided by scientific and public attitudes. The decisions of the present and future have yet to be made. Relevant values and scientific questions can only be resolved by examining the available possibilities.

If the scientific community cannot decide how to view madness; if society is not convinced that madness is a public problem; and if, in practice, patients are stored and ignored, the current outlook is indeed uncertain and perplexing.

3

normality-
abnormality:
by what
criterion

Popular books and articles about abnormal psychology generally convey the notion that abnormality is a fairly clear-cut thing; something one either does or does not have. Radio and television portray mental health as a carburetor that may get dirty or out of adjustment, but which may be readily repaired by a mental health expert. This presentation of mental illness implies that emotions, like any machine, may be adjusted or tuned-up. This is furthermore a reflection of the American ethos, the elevation of technology.

Abnormal texts usually list three major types of mental illness: *neuroses,* in which the person continues to function but is unhappy, inefficient, and maladaptive; *psychoses,* in which the person can no longer function and behaves in bizarre ways; and *character disorders,* in which the person behaves in such an irresponsible way with respect to others that something must be done about the person, for the sake of others. Each of these three categories has a variety of subtypes, and many of them have further subtypes. The symptoms of each are listed as a precise number of distinctively different entities, just as travel by air, land, and water are distinctively different, with each mode having its own specific subtypes of vehicles.

A deliberate effort will be made in this book to give a different picture of mental illness. There are many possible viewpoints for the identification of abnormality. Therefore, the nature of the phenomenon will be distorted by the notions used, and it will take different forms depending on which viewpoint is accepted.

When we say, in everyday language, that "Joe is normal" or "John is abnormal," we really mean that Joe fits our perception of what is normal and John, in our perception, acts strangely at times and does unusual things. But actions are not the only grounds for these labels. Often, it would be well-nigh impossible to list all the acts people consider abnormal. What it really boils down to is a belief that the person himself is strange.

The term "abnormality" roughly encompasses both the behavior the person exhibits and his or her personality. Traditionally, psychiatric judgments of normality and abnormality have depended more on the personality of the individual than on his behavior. Concern has been with what makes him tick, that is, with what is going on "inside," and indicates that it is John who is abnormal, not his behavior.

The focus on the personality of an individual might seem obvious because it reflects customary beliefs. Dynamic approaches to human behavior, like the psychoanalytic theory of Freud and his followers, have been concerned with the elements and the processes that make up the personality of the subject. Behavior as a basis for determining abnormality was largely ignored until recently.

A distinction between personality and behavior should be made. For example, if conditions of normality-abnormality are characteristics that operate inside the organism (personality), they are not directly observable. Such characteristics cannot be measured directly; therefore, the validity of the concepts must be inferred. Love or resentment towards one's mother must be inferred, for it is an attitude of the person, not a behavior. Such an attitude is an invention, created by the therapist, placed inside the person, and assumed to be useful in understanding him or her.

Judging from current theories of personality and mental illness, psychologists and psychiatrists have felt that the concept of personality was crucial and necessary. Behavior was considered a by-product of the personality.

Why the term "personality"?

The behavior of our close friends seldom surprises us. They do the things we expect them to do. They behave in much the same manner from day to day; in short, there is a certain consistency in their lives. Their behavior can be predicted. For example, consider three common types found on most college campuses.

The worrier is upset before every examination; he is convinced that he will do poorly, and exhibits signs of distress. He complains to his friends and to anyone who will listen that he is all washed up; finished; through. When the results are in, he is on top where he usually is; the predicted disaster never materializes.

Then there is the procrastinator, who never gets

around to studying or completing his work on time due to circumstances "beyond his control." His performance is poor but he can always proclaim that it doesn't really count because he didn't have a chance to show his real stuff; but just wait till next time.

And finally there is super hero who always plans his time and balances the effort expended on the various pressures, while still allowing some time for personal pleasure. On each and every examination he is prepared to the maximum possible without slighting other demands, and the result is equal to his highest potential.

Each of these three idealized types shows consistency; each approaches examinations demonstrating the same repeating pattern. Once such predictable behavior has been identified, it can be named and used to describe the behavior of other people. Hypotheses can then be developed to explain the origins of the behaviors. All people may then be seen as made up of sets of such behavioral characteristics—personality—which provide the basis for understanding their actions.

How consistent behavior may be used as a conceptual framework follows: the first two college students protected themselves against failure. The worrier, by loudly proclaiming he would fail, has already predicted and explained the reasons for the failure. If he does indeed fail, he need make no new excuses. A failure merely confirms the validity of that person's statement. The procrastinator always has an excuse for his failure, for he never puts himself to the test.

If we got a group of worriers together, we might discover that their parents had always demanded explanations: "Why did you spill your paint?" "Why did you wear your blue rather than green shirt?" "Why don't you color that dark green instead of light green? I certainly would!" Such questions imply disapproval. We might expect the worriers to see the world as a place where you always have to justify what you do. To be safe from disapproval—and from not being loved—this person must have an explanation for any performance that might be questioned.

People who procrastinated were afraid to try, we reason, and we might also discover that their parents treated them as irresponsible people, by making major and minor decisions for them and by disapproving of their independent actions, well into adolescence. The procrastinators continue to avoid responsibility for independent action because they cannot risk the possibility of confirming their inadequacy. A fear of responsible, self-initiated performance keeps them from risking maximum effort; if you haven't allowed your best effort to be evaluated, you cannot fail as a person.

The third student presumably had parents who loved him as a child, and he felt safe to try new, independent activities and accept greater responsibility for his decisions. He grew up in an atmosphere which was supportive of his independence and growth. The result was a person who could realistically appraise himself as well as the situation and act accordingly.

If people are to be described and understood in terms of their personality, their behavior traits must be true of people in general. A commitment to the concept of personality means in part that one is searching for a set of concepts to explain the consistencies in the behavior of many different people. These concepts must not be restricted to an individual but must be useful for predicting the behavior of many persons. The inner dispositions become the elements and dimensions used to describe, understand, and predict behavior.

The preceding statements about personality are not incontrovertible facts. People have personalities only if you are willing to view man in this way. Many mental health workers, therapists, and individuals concerned with abnormal behavior and with people in general, have been convinced that the idea of personality is a good one. But there is another point of view. In this book it is called *behavioral* and it will be presented as an alternate approach of general experimental psychology to the study of personality.

In summary: (1) There are consistencies in the behavior of a given individual over a period of time and between different people at any given time. Presumably these consistencies are the result of something. At this point the term "personality" is introduced as a way to account for consistencies. Thus, personality is a concept; it is a collection of characteristics and attributes that are inside an individual, and are used as the elements that determine current behavior. (2) From the personality point of view, these elements can be used to describe a healthy organism; when the correct value of each element has been ascertained, the individual is not only described, but the nature of his consistencies is known, for it is his personality which underlies his behaviors.

The personality approach has great economy, because each person does not have to be considered as unique. By describing personality in terms of these general elements, one can anticipate behavior. Personality provides a general way to understand man.

Another aspect of personality is that the consistencies tend to be self-sustaining. Our lifestyles have a way of eliciting congruent behavior from the world. Furthermore, our consistencies guide our perceptions and provide the dimensions we use to see, to explain, and to understand the behavior of those around us. If you are convinced that people are happy and that they do nice things for each other, you can elicit as well as notice this behavior. On the other hand, if you think people are disreputable and untrustworthy, they will act similarly toward you. You may find some ulterior motive behind everything—even something nice that is done for someone—thus confirming what an underhanded person the actor is.

Our beliefs, no less than scientific theories, define an event as one kind (such as friendly) rather than another (such as underhanded) on the basis of our assumptions. The same process holds for other events and distinctions made about them such as normal versus abnormal, or devil-ridden versus sick.

What has been said about personality can be applied to other aspects of living that are taken to be signs of normality or abnormality. The "it-is-a-nice world" perception is judged proper, and others are judged to be distorted. Such an approach moves us toward specifying what is a normal personality and what is an abnormal personality. But note that this requires a value judgment. It requires agreement about what is good and what is not. So far that decision has been too easy to make. The examples given above were set up to show how a notion of personality is related to the normal-abnormal distinction. A more complicated illustration will be useful to focus on the value judgment.

Take the example of Clara, from the film *The Feeling of Hostility,* produced by the National Film Board of Canada. Her father was killed when she was four. Her mother, in her grief, drew Clara very close to her, only to remarry when Clara was eleven or twelve. Clara felt deserted when the exceedingly close relationship between her and her mother was interrupted by the remarriage and then by the arrival of a baby brother. Clara was intellectually gifted, but this trait was exploited by her mother. Clara's report card was for exhibition; apparently she was not appreciated as a person, only her achievements were. Clara excelled in high school and college, but had developed a distrust of close interpersonal relationships. Clara expected other persons, based on her experience with her mother, to let her down and to use her. Achievement was a safe way to win non-personal approval and respect. Its competitive nature kept others at a distance. Clara's lifestyle protected her from being close to others, and because her actions were self-maintaining, change was difficult. Her coldness would drive away anyone who came too close. It was impossible to have a spontaneous, warm relationship with Clara. Her social life was always formal and potential suitors few. Clara's critical power and her intellectual ability took her into a profession where she enjoyed success. She received an editorial job that put her critical power to good use. The story of Clara ends with the job a success, but the evenings spent alone in her room. She is not happy, but she is not unhappy. She has a consistent way of living. Her lifestyle enables her to function well on her job and to be successful in her chosen field of work, but it also assures that she will be without the companionship of other people. For her success, she pays the price of loneliness.

Several points are worth noting. The simplest is the additional illustration of consistent personality traits and how lifestyles influence day-to-day behavior. Behavior has continuity and tends to sustain itself.

Human behavior is sufficiently complex that it has seemed necessary to postulate characteristics, traits, and attributes that are inside a person. Often these are things that the person is unaware of. For example, Clara did not seem to realize that she made comments that drove other people away from her. Her loneliness was not a deliberate price she paid for her other successes; it was no choice at all, but a course of action forced on her by her circumstances. Rather, Clara felt lonely at times without knowing the cause or what to do about it.

One way to make sense of Clara's life is by knowing things about her personality. Her personality was made up of several elements. There was the need to excel in order to feel secure and valued as a person; there was the need to keep others from getting too close because they could hurt her or let her down; and there was also the need to avoid being dependent on others. Her behavior can be explained in terms of the elements which describe her personality.

By introducing personality in this way, a consideration of normal-abnormal has been widened beyond specific behaviors. Success in her work was achieved by Clara only at the expense of interpersonal relationships. Yet, these distinctions exist only by looking inside the person to consider him or her as well as the behavior.

Normality then has at least two aspects—*what we do and what we are.* In what way are these aspects combined, and by what criterion are the judgments to be made? Could Clara have done her work as well if she were a different kind of person? And if not, how do you weigh success, when its achievement excludes other satisfactions or even has negative outcomes? Can these distinctions be made on absolute grounds, or are they merely defined by social convention, appropriate for here and now but completely relative in the long term? Is the act of doing something nice for someone either good or bad, or does it depend upon whether it is perceived as friendly or not? Behavior is public and observable, but the knowledge of motives requires a description of the actor's personality in terms of concepts attributed to him. How are these concepts to be verified? Can we possibly understand human behavior without them?

What constitutes normality and abnormality?

This question cannot be answered simply or specifically. Any answer carries with it implicit assumptions. Since several answers are possible, each based on different assumptions, a distinction between normality and abnormality is never absolute, only relative.

A distinction between what an individual does and what he is, is not always clear. Closely related to that is the question of whether abnormality is structural or functional. A structural approach requires the use of concepts of inner dispositions and organizations of these dispositions. Abnormality, then, depends upon chronic and long-term conditions of individuals, whether or not they are functioning adequately or inadequately at any given time. An arrested (or dormant) abnormal structure could exist within a person even though the current functioning is not disrupted. The alternative viewpoint, a functional definition, treats abnormality as an acute disruption of the person either in terms of inner dispositions or in terms of his ongoing behavior.

An additional unresolved issue is what William Scott referred to as the unitary versus the specific nature of mental illness. [1] Mental illness can be considered a unitary characteristic of the organism, so that in some basic sense, all mentally ill persons have something in common. Conversely, mental illness can be viewed as only a term, one which artificially groups together basically different disorders. If mental illness has a unitary characteristic, then delinquency and a paranoid state are similar, and efforts of prevention, treatment, and research can be organized around one professional group. If, on the other hand, delinquency and paranoid states are conceptually distinct, it may be better to treat them quite differently.

40

Knowledge about mental illness, from the era of witchcraft to the present time, indicates that neither normality nor abnormality has an absolute meaning. Therefore, the definition is arbitrary. The issues of primary concern are the *assumptions* that are made about human nature that determine how a person is to be treated.

Mental patients who are committed to psychiatric hospitals are deprived of their civil liberties. Whether a person is sane or insane determines, for example, his ability to make a binding agreement and his standing before the law.

If you are quite content with your life, satisfied with what you are doing and the world in general, by what criteria are you willing to let others commit you to a psychiatric hospital? On what grounds are you willing to permit others to disregard what you say about your own happiness? Are you willing to let others examine the nature of your internal make up and arrive at a decision—apart from any specific behavior or acts that you may have committed—and decide that you are possessed with the devil or with mental illness?

Judgments about other people's mental health contain implicit moral and ethical standards. Our age is one of relativism; the culture is continually changing, so that what is correct now may not be correct in twenty, or ten, or even five years. Different cultures have different moral and ethical standards. What is normal in one culture may be abnormal in another. There is a certain fallacy in using ethical or moral standards even within a culture. Who has the right to decide which morals or ethics are to be followed? Is the success orientation—a hard-working, self-reliant, pioneer spirit so often held up as the spirit of Americanism—to be the only guide for mental health and normality? Is a personality that embodies these behaviors the personification of mental health?

The unanswered question is how much the moral and value judgments about abnormality are relative to a definite time and place. The question of normality is tied to conformity with the values of the time. But there is also a timeless criterion, an ideal for maximizing social adjustment that is distinct and separate from the values of the existing social order.

A case in point

The following incident was related to me by a colleague several years ago. The incident brings into focus some of the abstract issues which have been discussed.

A middle-aged woman was admitted to a psychiatric hospital in an acutely disturbed condition. She was delusional and hallucinated, living in a make-believe world of her own imagination. She believed that she had a child, which in fact she did not have. Her daily activities and her life focused on the care of this imaginary child. She talked to it; she fed it. She bathed her baby and bought it clothes. She did everything that a good mother should do for her child.

The patient's husband told the story. He was a janitor in a medium-sized, high-rise Chicago apartment building. He and his wife lived in a small, but comfortable, basement apartment. She kept the apartment clean and neat and took excellent care of their old, but adequate furniture.

The janitor and his wife were generally well-liked by the tenants in the building, and especially by the children, to whom they were both especially kind. He would fix their broken toys and would stop to talk with the children. The janitor took their concerns seriously. He was always patient and understanding whenever they watched or "helped" him repair things in their apartment. His wife frequently baked cookies for the children. The couple seemed happy.

The janitor and his wife truly enjoyed children, but as they grew older, they realized that they probably were not going to have any of their own. This was a great disappointment to them, but nevertheless, they made the best of it by the satisfaction they received from children in the building. On several occasions, they had tried to adopt children. However, they were of modest means and of a lower socio-economic class. Their living quarters were small and both had restricted educational backgrounds. Neither seemed particularly bright. All of this was enough to exclude the possibility of adopting a child from an agency.

Christmas was an especially difficult time for them. It was then they especially missed the child they would have liked to have had. On the very first Christmas after their marriage, they had taken the money from their penny jar and bought Christmas presents for some of the children in the building, especially those who were likely to receive few gifts. The night before Christmas they played Mr. and Mrs. Santa Claus while distributing gifts for the children. They continued to do this every year thereafter. This ritual became a big Christmas event for the couple. Their wants were small, and even though their income was modest, they had always managed to set aside some money each week in their penny jar. The couple derived great satisfaction from this tradition, especially on Christmas morning, when an excited child made a special trip to their apartment to show them what Santa had left.

At some point in this tradition, the janitor and his wife sort of pretended to be buying the toys for "their" child. And at another point, and it was hard to put an exact time on it, they were shopping for "their" child rather than for the children in the building. Of course, they distributed the toys as usual to the children in the building. But, one year, the janitor's wife thought it would be fun to hold back

43

one of the toys they had bought, to wrap it, and to keep it themselves just as if they were going to give it to their own child. After all, it could be used when the children visited, as they so often did.

Over a period of time, there was a little bit more make-believe and a little bit more pretending at Christmas time. Of course, it was always quite clear that they were just pretending. To them this was simply another way to get a little more satisfaction out of their lives and compensate for their disappointment. For the wife, however, the size of the pretending gradually became larger and larger. For example, one Christmas she suggested setting a place for their child at the Christmas dinner table. Then on later occasions she wanted to serve food to the child. From that point, the pretending grew faster and faster out of proportion. The pretend child was there on other days in addition to Christmas.

The disappointed woman also began to set a dinner place and prepare food for the child. It was only a small step to buying children's clothes, and finally talking to a child who was not there.

That was the story the husband told. He looked at the psychiatrist and asked: "Where did we go wrong, Doc? Was it wrong to want a child? Was it wrong for us to buy Christmas presents for the children in the building? Was it wrong for us to sort of pretend we were really buying them for our child? I did it, too! Was it wrong to set a dinner place at the Christmas table? Is that where we went wrong, Doc? Is that the place where we should have quit pretending?"

How are such questions to be answered? Is it abnormal to buy Christmas presents for a child that you would like to have had, knowing full well that you are going to give them to other children? Should one consider it abnormal or mentally ill for that couple to do those things for the children in the building? Many would find their actions touching and

44

admirable. Was the behavior of setting a place at the dinner table only on Christmas Day an abnormal act? In a sense, it was certainly unusual and not in keeping with the reality of the situation, but, on the other hand, it provided some satisfaction by filling a void the couple felt in their life. Is this healthy or not? We all do this kind of thing to a certain extent, frequently with good results, by satisfying a want in an indirect way when a direct satisfaction is not available.

Perhaps a personality description of these two individuals is in order to decide how normal or abnormal their behavior was. This requires a conceptualization of their inner dispositions to discover what might be motivating their behavior. On these grounds, toy-buying might be judged healthy and normal for the man because it was a reasonable way of satisfying one of his desires, but not for his wife for whom it was a distortion of reality, motivated by the wrong reasons. If you are willing to entertain the idea that this is possible, then the importance of inner dispositions in discussing what is normal and abnormal has been illustrated.

The wife's difficulty can be seen as a structural weakness in her personality, so that the chronic state of pretending eventually took over her life. A different explanation approaches her breakdown as an acute state. For this view, the idea of abnormality is meaningful only in terms of her current or acute behavior.

The unitary versus the specific nature of abnormality is concerned with whether or not this woman is similar to a delinquent. Are the concepts used to understand her also the ones needed to understand the delinquent? At the practical level, the question is whether or not the mental health movement should be addressed to both, and if so, if the basis for confinement and treatment are to be derived from common concepts.

In this case, the woman was soon relieved of her

delusions by electric shock treatment and discharged from the hospital much improved. However, her disappointment regarding children was never resolved and the aura of fun that had been part of their lives for many years at Christmas time was gone forever. The chance for permanent recovery in such cases is not good. She might well return, but the information will exist only as an entry in some statistical summary of readmission rates.

4

the
nature
of
explanation

At this point it is important to have a clear understanding of what it means to explain human behavior. Different concepts have been used to label and explain unusual behavior. One concept is known historically as madness, but in current terms, the behavior is called mental illness. Both describe the same kind of human behavior. Concepts provide an explanation by specifying how some event is to be seen and what information and knowledge is relevant. There are two important and related aspects of concepts. One consideration is the problem created when there is more than one way to explain something. The second aspect is how the concepts themselves are to be viewed (which requires having concepts about concepts).

Levels of explanation

Consider juvenile delinquency as an example. From a sociological point of view, one might assume that a particular kind of neighborhood produces delinquency. A concept such as social disorganization could be used to explain it. From this point of view, delinquency would be expected more frequently in a low-rent district, where there is lack of education, impoverishment, and many broken homes. The delinquent behavior is explained in terms of some form of social disorganization.

Now, consider delinquency using a social-psychological approach. This explanation is based on studies of peer group behavior. This implies that the juvenile delinquent learns his antisocial code of behavior from his peers. This peer sanctioned behavior assures his status and acceptance as a person within the group. He engages in delinquent acts as a result of the group and its demands.

A psychological interpretation of juvenile delinquency studies the individual himself for an explanation of why he is delinquent. It may be pointed out, for example, that he was criticized and beaten at home and that he feels inferior. As a result of these personal experiences, he is motivated to seek power to compensate for and overcome a deep sense of personal weakness. Those needs for power are satisfied by defying authority, by stealing cars, and by the psychological feeling gained from taking risks. The delinquent behavior is a form of psychological compensation.

Thus far, delinquent behavior has been given three different levels of explanation. Which is the right way to describe and explain the behavior? The answer is that behavior owes no allegiance to any particular theoretical explanation. Rather, any particular bit of behavior may be explained in many different ways, and from many different approaches to the problem. All of the different levels of explanation are potentially valid and useful.

For example, in the case of juvenile delinquency, if one were interested in city renovation, or if one were a member of a city-planning commission for urban renewal, the sociological interpretation of juvenile delinquency would be appropriate, the best theoretical explanation. This knowledge could aid the task of planning so as to combat or minimize various forms of social disorganization. The effectiveness of the plan would depend both on the usefulness of the theory and on the adequacy of the particular courses of action that were derived from the theory.

If a person was a director of a youth center, he or she might be primarily interested in a social-psychological explanation of delinquency. For this purpose, it would be well to know how to change the values of the peer group. It would be useful to understand how group processes operate so that he or she would know how to combat or to deal with the roots of delinquency. The success of the effort would depend in part on the power of the theory and what particular courses of action from the theory were carried out.

On the other hand, a psychotherapist interested in changing the behavior of one particular delinquent, or a parole officer trying to help particular individuals, might be more interested in an individual or psychological explanation. They might be interested in knowing more about the individual personality of a boy to understand his specific psychological needs, or to ascertain forces that are operating to motivate him to behave in such a manner. An explanation of these inner feelings might be most useful, for they concern the psychological processes that determined his behavior. Success would depend, in part, on the adequacy of the theory; whether or not one correctly attributed the proper characteristics to the individual, and how appropriately one planned and effected particular concrete courses of action.

Put more simply, *particular events owe no allegiance to any particular level of explanation*, or for that matter, to any particular theoretical point of view. An event—an observable bit of behavior—does not intrinsically prove or disprove any theoretical point of view. Events themselves are only interpretable. Events form the basis from which inferences are drawn. The inference itself will be more or less useful for some given, but limited, purpose. The usefulness of any particular level of explanation is always related to some purpose or goal, and is also relative to the state of knowledge that exists at any given time. Any theoretical explanation of behavior may also be discarded at any time. The state of knowledge is always relative; a new or a better theoretical explanation may appear to replace the present one. The events, the facts, the observables of behavior do not change; however, the system of explanation or of inferences that have been abstracted change. In this way, any theoretical point of view must be considered as an invention, which may be used where applicable.

Personality and psychopathology are especially open to different levels of explanation. The relative power of different levels of explanation is not often directly open to evaluation, partly because the criterion is remote and because there are other considerations that go beyond the explanation itself. For example, would a city planner's failure to prevent social disorganization discredit a sociological explanation of delinquency? Would the failure of parole officers to deal with delinquent boys discredit a psychological approach to human processes? In both cases, the reason for the failure could be due to inadequate understanding or implementation as well as other external factors.

Explanations about deviant behavior are closed to direct evaluation for still another reason. Interpretations are usually at different levels of abstraction, and the implications are not strictly comparable. Of course, the empirical and practical consequences ultimately define how useful theories are, where and how they work, and for what. But choosing between alternative approaches is a difficult, slow, continual, and somewhat arbitrary process, much as was the process of switching from devils to illness as a suitable explanation of madness. Changing from current concepts to future ones may also be difficult.

The field of abnormal psychology currently is in a stage of turmoil and ferment. The problems of mental health are pressing. The practical consequences of various explanations are weak and vague and the range of their usefulness has been hard to determine. Theories which approach mental health and illness at different levels with little common ground on which to compare them, are the cause of much contention between their proponents.

Then, too, one cannot discount the fact that mental health practitioners have a direct economic and personal stake in choosing one theory over another. The struggle itself is important because new views are emerging. But this is just the beginning. At this point, the study of abnormal psychology is as much a matter of deciding what it is as inventing ways to understand it. Some differences among various theoretical explanations of mental illness are caused by different notions of what it is. We have seen some gross examples of this, and there are more subtle illustrations of this later on.

Multiple Determinism

Another approach to an explanation of abnormal behavior is to say that events have multiple causes. An event does not have a single cause. In this sense, there are different causes, or explanations, for the occurrence of the behavior.

Unfortunately, psychological theories of human behavior are still weak and diffuse. Not one is universally accepted, even as an explanation of the most simple behavioral phenomenon. The lack of powerful psychological concepts is inevitable, because of the short history of the behavioral sciences. The idea that man could be studied scientifically and the commitment of resources toward this goal have lagged considerably behind the earlier equally unpopular idea—that nature could be studied scientifically. The central point is that we invent our explanations, and only in this sense are there causes. It is a matter of definition. In principle, the same event can have an endless stream of causes. In psychology this is also true; and in psychology there are no theories so powerful as to render competitive theoretical inventions impotent.

5

the diagnostic system

Most textbooks of abnormal psychology refer to three major kinds of mental illnesses: character disorders, neuroses, and psychoses. These are general classifications and each is broken down into several different types and subcategories. For example, the psychoses are typically divided into four subcategories: schizophrenia, paranoia, affective reactions, and involutional psychotic reactions. These various subheadings may be further divided. For example, schizophrenia is one kind of psychosis, but it is diagnostically divided into four main types: simple, hebephrenic, catatonic, and paranoid, plus several other lesser categories. In this chapter we will consider these four subvarieties. Our primary interest, however, will not be to communicate information about schizophrenia; this particular disorder merely serves as a focal point and provides the illustrative material for a discussion about diagnosis in general. We will be primarily concerned with the nature of the diagnostic system and the purposes that it serves.

Schizophrenia, as one of the most incapacitating forms of mental illness, is one of the most urgent problems of psychopathology. Schizophrenic patients occupy more hospital beds than patients with any other single type of psychiatric disorder. They accumulate in hospitals because the prognosis for recovery is poor.

The simple schizophrenic shows a general reduction of interest, very shallow human relationships marked by a lack of interest in other people, and affectively, is apathetic and indifferent to all that surrounds him or her. That picture may be contrasted with the hebephrenic type; this individual makes silly, inappropriate, and stereotyped emotional responses. The gestures and activities are generally inappropriate to the situation and are primarily composed of repetitive mannerisms. Paranoid schizophrenics, on the other hand, frequently have delusions and hallucinations. They often believe that they are in great danger and that other people are conniving against them. At times, paranoid schizophrenics are aggressive and hostile. The catatonic types show very conspicuous motor behavior; these people are either very inhibited or hyperactive. On one occasion, there may be a very marked display of motor activity in catatonic schizophrenics, and on other occasions, there is complete inhibition of any motor response. This inhibition has been called "waxy flexibility," which simply means that another person can move or place the catatonic's arms in a new position, and he or she will leave them there.

Why should these four seemingly very different

patterns of symptoms be grouped together under a general heading of schizophrenia? By what principle can one say that the simple, the hebephrenic, the paranoid, and the catatonic type all belong to a single general class of disorders? Some psychologists and psychiatrists think there is a justification for grouping them together; others do not. Some of the general characteristics which have been proposed as a basis for grouping the categories together are: (1) all four types show a marked incapacity to evaluate reality, and consequently their relationships with other people are disturbed; (2) there is a disorganization of both thought processes and emotions. The disorganization in its intellectual form shows as a loss of the ability to think abstractly and conceptually. In its social form, there is a loss of role-playing skills and an inability to interact affectively with other people. These two aspects, the lack of contact with reality and the conceptual and social disorganization, are used to justify grouping the four categories together as specific manifestations of a common disorder called schizophrenia. Such a proposal needs to be re-evaluated.

A Descriptive Taxonomy

Let us stop for a moment to consider the implications of such a diagnostic system and what it can tell us about diagnosis in general. The outstanding feature of diagnosis lies in the fact that it is a descriptive system only. The categories have been invented (not discovered) by looking at the behavior of patients and then abstracting from this behavior what is felt to be its essential features. Once these have been identified descriptively, a set of principles or abstractions is found which allows one to group some of them together to form categories or types. In short, a diagnostic system is an attempt to build a set of ideas or concepts that will allow others to sort out various behaviors that are seen clinically and to classify them into their appropriate types.

It is the same process as sorting a bunch of objects and placing them in categories. One could sort them, for example, on the basis of color; putting the red ones in one pile, the blue in another, the green and the yellow in still other piles. When finished, there would be a classification system based on color, and any new items could be sorted into one of the four different categories, more or less accurately, depending on the hues and brightnesses of the objects. All of the objects in one category would be more or less alike with respect to one characteristic they all share—color. Any one of the objects in any one of the piles might be made of different materials, have variations in volume, shape, thickness, or weight, and could differ on any number of additional characteristics.

The simple example of sorting objects may be used to illustrate what has been done with the various kinds of behavior pathology. For example, our diagnostic system historically comes largely from the work of Kraepelin, who observed mental patients over a long period of time, and by observing them, selected certain elements to arrive at a classification system. He hoped that by careful descriptions, he could invent a classification system to group together the patients with a similar etiology. The classification could aid ostensibly in identifying the underlying cause more quickly.

A descriptive diagnostic system is in use in psychiatry today. It is an extension and purification of the Kraepelin system. The very different symptomatology of simple, hebephrenic, paranoid, and catatonic schizophrenics are grouped together as common forms of one disorder. They are grouped together on the proposition that they are similar with respect to withdrawal from reality and manifestations of social and intellectual disorganization.

It is an article of faith that a descriptive system will be useful for isolating antecedent conditions and developing different treatment techniques. However, there are important differences between the descriptive system used for mental illness, and those used for other illnesses. For example, classifying a case as tubercular carries some fairly specific implications. For one thing, it means that a particular infectious agent can be found in the lungs of the individual. It means that the disorder will follow a fairly specific course, and that a relatively consistent set of symptoms will occur over the term of the illness. Likewise, it is known that rest and other treatment techniques can terminate or alleviate the disorder. The treatment for tuberculosis is different from the treatment given to a patient with a persistent cough that is the aftermath of a common cold or excessive smoking. The diagnosis in this case implies different treatment.

Specific information is known about many common illnesses. The diagnostic label tells something about antecedent conditions, the probable course of the illness, the symptoms that will occur, and the treatment to be given. Of course, even this information is relative. New treatment techniques are continually devised and more sensitive diagnostic procedures developed to differentiate between two symptomatically similar, but etiologically different, disorders. New information about the biology and biochemistry of human organisms will offer the possibility of new and more powerful ways to prescribe the treatment for various illnesses.

Contrast this kind of diagnosis with that used in psychiatry today. Mental disorders have not, as yet, been shown to be of a similar nature. The etiological agents are unknown, the course of the mental disorder is unreliable, and differential treatment techniques do not follow uniformly from specific diagnosis. However, several treatment procedures, such as electric shock, are more likely to be used with some disorders than others. But the extent to which they are effective is an empirical observation, a technological feat unfounded in theoretical understanding of the particular disorder.

There are various and conflicting viewpoints on the nature of schizophrenia. There are those who argue for a psychological interpretation of the etiology of schizophrenia, those who emphasize heredity, and others who emphasize biochemical make-up. When someone is called a "schizophrenic," the label is of a different type than that of general paresis. When someone is called a schizophrenic, there is no assurance that the label conveys information about the antecedent conditions, either on a psychological, hereditary, or biochemical level. Indeed, it is not certain that a patient would be diagnosed in the same way in a different psychiatric hospital. Not only psychiatric diagnosis, but also the symptoms the patient shows are unreliable. On one day a patient may look more like a hebephrenic type of schizophrenic and on the next day more like a simple type. Patients do not show the classic symptomatology of each of the subtypes described in textbooks. The classic case is the exception rather than the rule. Classic cases are immediately placed before the hospital staff in a case conference because of their illustrative value.

The meaning of the four subtypes of schizophrenia is open to various interpretations by various people using various levels of explanation. Nothing in the diagnosis by subtypes will allow one to specify how or when or why the disorder will terminate. Some patients get better and some don't. Some of those discharged from the hospital are able to live full lives and some cannot. Others suffer remissions and come back to the hospital. Remission seems to occur for all categories of schizophrenia.

What is the fundamental value of a diagnosis based on a descriptive system which carries little information either about the etiology or the course of the illness? An important reason for any diagnosis is that it provides one way to look for antecedent conditions so as to determine the proper treatment. Diagnosis implies that dividing the patient population into subgroups on the basis of common characteristics will yield ways to determine the causes and courses of various disorders.

Remember the illustration given earlier about sorting different objects on the basis of color? The objects were placed in red, blue, green, and yellow piles, even though they had different shapes and sizes and were made of different materials. But, someone else could sort these objects in a different way by putting all of the wooden ones together, paper ones in another pile, iron in a third pile, and plastic objects in a fourth. Now they are grouped according to material contents. This sorting represents a different idea about the fundamental basis of classification. The new system can now be used to classify other objects. Indeed, both systems could be tried on another set of objects to see which one was most efficient or more reliable. A classification system is an arbitrary scheme that is applied to objects for particular purposes. Any one system might be more or less easy to use and more or less useful for some given purpose.

The problems illustrated above can be generalized to the process of psychiatric diagnosis. Ordinarily there is a complex, confusing mass of data and information about patients and their symptoms which can be categorized and dealt with in many different ways. Just because certain people are classified first as psychotic, then as schizophrenic, which can be further subdivided, does not mean that this is the correct method. It is an arbitrary decision. How useful this particular method will prove to be is an empirical question, a question for which currently there is no clear answer. Intrinsically, there is nothing right or wrong about any diagnostic system. There can, of course, be things wrong from a practical point of view. The field of mental disorders is wide open enough so that anyone could come along and examine the array of symptoms and behaviors and invent some new set of ideas. I do not mean to imply that the task is easy or even that it is a wise undertaking. Apparently many psychologists and psychiatrists feel that the current system is on the right track. The essential point is that the diagnostic procedure is an arbitrary one and may be more or less useful than some other system not yet specified. The state of knowledge is such that room always exists for competitive systems of ideas.

The discussion so far has been kept on a fairly simple level. In point of fact, descriptive diagnostic systems can be extremely complex. To use the previous example, one could retain the original grouping of color and further divide the objects on the basis of the type of material, either wood, plastic, metal, or paper. Such a multiple classification would be a more complex system, but it could be done in many ways. For example, the material could be made the primary basis for the distinction and the color of the material could then be a subclassification. In using a two-dimensional classification system, we have ignored other characteristics and other concepts that could have been applied to the objects. The objects might have been divided further on the basis of shape (squares, circles, triangles, and rectangles), by height, weight, the design on the face of the object, texture, and so forth. The problem is to decide which similarities should be ignored. Surely it is more efficient to ignore some characteristics of the objects and use others as the basis for classification.

The analogy can be applied to mental disorders.

We can hardly use a diagnostic system that is so complex and has so many dimensions that only one or two people belong in each category. We need concepts which isolate cases having certain common antecedent conditions, common courses, or respond differentially to various treatments. We have to select the most salient dimensions and ignore the dimensions that are irrelevant for the purposes of understanding and managing individual cases. Refining concepts, subtle shifting of categories, and selecting criteria must be a never-ending process if more useful concepts are to be invented. At the present time, we are in a most gross stage of this refinement.

The whole point of this discussion can be illustrated by reviewing a small and selected sample of the research that has been done on schizophrenia. It will illustrate the arbitrary nature of diagnosis, the value and the limitations of such systems, and the progress, refinement, and clarification that takes place over time as we become better able to organize events into a more comprehensive arbitrary system.

Many psychiatrists and psychologists believe that the concepts of withdrawal from reality and the social and intellectual disorganization taken together reflect the fundamental nature of a unitary disorder called schizophrenia, which may be further divided into four types on the basis of secondary symptoms. Thus, out of the wide variety of symptom patterns shown by patients in general, four "objects" have been separated from the rest and called schizophrenia.

We could ignore the differences among the types and call them irrelevant, and then there would be no need for the distinction. These differences, however, have not been ignored. A great deal of research has attempted to account for them. It is reasonable to assume that different kinds of experience or different personality traits exist for each of the forms of schizophrenia. It is also natural to assume that the four types will have a different prognosis for recovery or they will respond differentially to different kinds of treatment. This is a reasonable way for research to proceed. Information, facts, and events are discovered, but our interpretations of them, our concepts, theories, and laws are invented. In the case of the diagnostic system, they were passed by popular vote. The official labels, the number and varieties of subtypes of various disorders, were elected to their place in the *Diagnostic and Statistical Manual of Mental Disorders* written and approved by members of the American Psychiatric Association.[1] This further illustrates the arbitrary nature of the system by which we view mental illness.

Schizophrenia

Tasks of intellectual and cognitive functioning have existed for a number of years, and it was only natural that they would be applied to schizophrenics as well as other patients. One of the distinguishing features of psychiatric patients is low scores on tasks requiring reasoning and concept formation. This deficit has been observed in schizophrenics for some time, as illustrated by the old term *dementia praecox* which was based on a presumed organic deterioration after adolescence. The more neutral term of "psychological deficit," has come into use recently; this new term merely indicates poor performance on intellectual tasks without assuming a deteriorating organic basis of the decrement. If schizophrenia is a unitary disorder, it is reasonable to predict that schizophrenics would show a similarity in cognitive deficits. In a thorough review of this research, one psychiatrist concluded that: "Schizophrenics in general are so heterogeneous that there is no real reason to regard them as suffering from a single disease entity."[2] From the performance of schizophrenics on cognitive tasks, it is not clear that the group shows any consistent type of performance clearly responsible for their psychological deficit.

But other researchers have conceptualized the psychological deficit shown by schizophrenics on cognitive tasks differently. They were able to show that the types of errors made by schizophrenics were different from those shown by patients with known brain damage or from those caused by the organic deterioration which occurs with age. Furthermore, the hypothesis was advanced that the uneven performance by schizophrenics occurred because they were especially sensitive to threats of criticism and rebuff that are present in social situations. It was proposed that this sensitivity was responsible for their poor performance. In this context the psychological deficit can be viewed as a motivational problem.

The study of the family backgrounds of schizophrenics further supports the notion that their motivational defect does indeed reflect a sensitivity to censure particularly as a consequence of never being able to satisfy the expectations of their mothers. The results of early research generated by this motivational view were positive. For example, if schizophrenics were censured for errors by the word, "wrong," their performance got worse, while normals would try harder and do better. However, the results were not always consistent and sometimes censure produced better, rather than worse, performance; and praise and positive reinforcement were not always effective in facilitating performance. The responsiveness of schizophrenics to praise in a supportive, noncritical context was taken to be consistent with censure hypothesis, since the removal of interpersonal stress should reduce the psychological deficit.

Inconsistent and sometimes contradictory findings were common here, however, and the validity of the hypothesis has been hard to evaluate. For example, how much support and praise does the experimenter have to give in order to overcome the schizophrenic's sensitivity to criticism? Does a negative finding reflect on the experimenter's failure to be sufficiently supporting or on the hypothesis itself?

Analysis by subtypes was of little help in clearing up the confusion about similarities of schizophrenic patients. However, investigation of their family backgrounds led to some new ideas. For example, in some cases, schizophrenics showed signs of interpersonal stress and isolation from other people early in their premorbid history. Other patients had a more normal premorbid period and a rather sudden onset of the disorder. These two types were labeled "poor" and "good" premorbid schizophrenics. It was found that the poor premorbids (also called process schizophrenics) had a poorer prognosis for recovery and were likely to become chronic patients. On the other hand, the good premorbids (also called reactive schizophrenics) had a better chance of recovery and were more likely to be in an acute and disturbed state.

This new way to subdivide schizophrenia into two rather than four types had value other than predicting prognosis. The poor premorbid patients were seen as motivated primarily by the desire to avoid censure, while the good premorbids, with their more normal backgrounds, were still amenable to positive reinforcement such as praise. This distinction helped explain why praise and censure did not always have the anticipated results in some research studies. Consequently, it became necessary to consider the premorbid history. Still, certain inconsistent and contradictory findings remained.

A doctoral dissertation by Louise Irwin done under this investigator's supervision can be used as an illustration of how conceptual systems are extended bit by bit.[3]We proposed a scheme that would explain the contradictory findings, indicating the conditions under which a deficit would or would not occur. We reasoned that if schizophrenics with a bad premorbid adjustment were primarily motivated to avoid censure, there would be no deficit if the censure could best be avoided by giving the correct answer. To test our idea, we asked a series of questions over and over again as many as fifteen times until the subject gave all correct responses. On one occasion, we used a simple task in which each of the questions had only two possible answers, one correct and one incorrect. Therefore, either answer gave the patient complete knowledge about what he should answer in the next round of questions. On this task we did not expect the bad premorbids to show an intellectual deficit because the censure could be avoided by giving the correct response.

However, on another occasion, the patients were given a more complex task in which there were eight possible responses; therefore, the censure of wrong for any particular mistake did not provide the subject with the correct answers for the following session. Under the stress of censure, we thought, schizophrenic symptoms would be brought out and an intellectual deficit should occur.

Also, because the poor premorbids are clinically assumed to be relatively indifferent to praise, it would not be a positive reinforcement and their performance would not be improved by its use. On the other hand, the good premorbids were expected to be influenced by praise because of their more normal family backgrounds and (unlike the poor premorbids) do better on the simple task with praise, and be less upset by censure on the complex task.

In statistical terms, an interaction was expected between the type of reinforcement (praise or censure), task complexity (simple or complex), and premorbid adjustment (good or bad). In our study, empirical support was obtained for our scheme by explaining how all three of these factors are related to whether or not an intellectual deficit exists in schizophrenic patients. The process of conceptualization, experimentation, and conceptual refinement is a never-ending circle.

Unfortunately, schizophrenia is not as clear-cut as it has heretofore been described. Not all persons with a pathogenic family background for schizophrenia will become schizophrenics or even patients, and of those who do become patients, not all will be schizophrenics. And, some who are schizophrenics will have normal backgrounds.

The research results reported here are only trends, because additional unknown factors play a role and because the family data are not free from error. The information gained about family history could have been a result of the questions asked, rather than something objectively observed. It is easy to find what we are looking for when we know what we want to find. Also, because the information is retrospective, we cannot be sure it is accurate.

Considerable time and effort is spent studying the parents and the family situations of schizophrenics to ascertain, if possible, what influence they may have had on the patients. However, in seeking answers from the parents to extremely detailed questions, we must assume their answers might well be incomplete or inconclusive. Remembering in great detail events that happened in the past is difficult for anyone.

In one investigation, regular interviews were held with mothers beginning immediately after the birth of their child to determine and record the child's development. The experimenters then made periodic observations of the child at home to establish the accuracy of the report. In as short a span as three years, most mothers were unable to remember with even reasonable accuracy when their child did what; and the occurrence of actual problem behavior was forgotten. Selective remembering occurred with middle-class mothers who were more likely to observe their children's development carefully; who had already reported these things as they occurred; and who knew the experimenter to be keeping a record. Who can say what distortions may occur through selective recall when a schizophrenic's parent tries to report on his childhood and family life to an investigator?[4]

The picture is further clouded by the existence of other theories to explain many of the same empirical results. By using different assumptions, these theories provide alternate pictures of the nature of schizophrenia; ones which imply other types of causes. A lucid account of the struggle to find meaning about a disorder as bizarre as schizophrenia is presented by psychologist Arnold Buss in his book, *Psychopathology*.[5] Buss suggests the disorder is inherited and posits that the study of genetic factors could be the central focus of research. He emphasizes biochemical factors and suggests the possibility of pharmacological solutions. In each case the evidence is suggestive, but inconclusive because of methodological difficulties similar to the family background and case history collation problems discussed here.

The point of this material on schizophrenia is to illustrate the arbitrary nature of our classification system. A helpful scheme for one problem may not make sense when viewed from the demands presented by a different problem. This has been illustrated by the failure of a classification based on symptoms to be related to the nature of cognitive deficits. The adequacy of cognitive functioning was clarified, however, by a consideration of motivational characteristics and a further subdivision in two categories based on premorbid history. Experiments do not *prove* anything. They provide an event which is only considered important because of the way it may be interpreted.

We have a descriptive diagnostic system. To call someone a neurotic, a psychotic, a schizophrenic, or a particular type of schizophrenic means next to nothing at this point. It does tell a few things about the person's symptoms. The label is of little value in dictating the type of treatment to be given, the course the illness follows, or its eventual outcome. A catatonic schizophrenic doesn't really exist. It may not be a reasonable term at all.

The diagnostic system we use is important, for it determines what conceptual pieces are available to be used for building our knowledge. A classification system may be valued from a research point of view for what new facts and subsequent ideas it can uncover. But beyond this, it has little value. We are using a set of invented ideas for classifying objects; the invention of the term schizophrenia, although still at a gross level, currently seems much better than the previous label of witchcraft.

6

mental illness
versus
behavior disorder

In the last chapter, it was shown that a particular diagnostic system is merely an interim set of hypotheses that can be used as a tool for progress. The mental health system, furthermore, is dissimilar to the system of labeling and classification which typically occurs in medicine. This, then, raises the question of whether we should refer to psychopathology as "mental illness," (a term which implies a disease viewpoint) or use a more neutral term such as "behavior disorder." The choice of one or the other is a matter of preference or belief rather than fact. The difference in terms, however, is fundamental, for it rests on a priori assumptions of how to conceptualize human behavior.

A distinction

Let us examine the difference between the two labels of madness. The traditional concept of an illness implies a set of symptoms, a specific etiology, and a specific treatment. In an infection, the body is invaded by an external agent which attacks an organ, may destroy tissue, or in some way disrupt the operation of the body. The symptoms reflect either the defensive operation of the body to protect itself or the consequences of an imperfectly functioning system (too much water retention resulting from kidney failure). The treatment is to rid the body of the infectious agent and restore balance or normality. Other illnesses result from the failure of some system or organ of the body, as in deterioration with age, and even when the cause of the malfunction is not clearly understood, the organ failure itself can be identified. In any case, the interdependence among systems and knowledge of their functions is specified in sufficient detail to permit understanding of the symptoms and the consequences of malfunction of one system on another. These organ failures and their consequences can be further examined at autopsy.

The knowledge of organ systems, their functions and interdependencies, does not always permit treatment; many malfunctions are not understood in the sense that their etiology cannot be specified, although their course usually can be specified. Others cannot be successfully treated, although something about the etiology is known. Not all damage is reparable. The central point is that organ malfunction, ways to produce it, ways to alleviate it, and its consequences are fairly well-known. It is in this broad category of bodily functioning that illness and disease occur.

To a certain extent, a parallel between the organic and psychopathological diseases can be established. Thus, if one talks about the failure of the organism to adapt to external and environmental attacks which disrupt its normal functioning, it makes little difference whether the stress is from the environment or from a germ. In either case, the organism has not adapted.

Therefore, protecting self-esteem may be seen as similar to the regulation of body water balance, for homeostasis is sought. In this broader sense, imbalance in both instances is similar and meets the definition of illness.

However, another important distinction must be made. A death caused by abnormal water balance leaves behind a diseased kidney to be inspected. But death (suicide) due to loss of self-esteem cannot be examined. The defective psychological system cannot be inspected. The concepts used to describe, to understand, to predict, and to control (organic) illnesses are very different from the concepts used for psychopathology.

Another distinction of psychopathology is its reliance on social values to define what madness is and what it is not. There are important practical differences that arise from the distinction between illness as a medical concept and behavior disorder as a social concept. These practical implications center on whether or not psychopathology is to remain in the province of medicine as an aid to solving health problems or is to be shifted to the area of behavior control, and considered an aid to solving social problems.

There are many psychologists who think the term "mental illness" is inappropriate, and that a better and more appropriate term is "behavior disorder." From our current concepts of psychopathology which emphasize the role of social and interpersonal factors, designation as behavior disorder is more appropriate. The definition of madness is to be found in both behavior and in

71

personality dispositions which deviate from social norms and values, but *not* as deviations from biological norms. A discussion of the social aspects of abnormal behavior suggests that the more neutral term "behavior disorder" may indeed offer a better conceptual framework than the label of mental illness.

Social aspects of madness

Psychiatrist Thomas Szasz has frequently and forcefully discussed these issues beginning in 1961 with his book *The Myth of Mental Illness*. Szasz makes it clear that he is not belittling the help that psychiatry can provide; but he is attempting to correct popular misconceptions about what psychiatry can and should do.[1] Szasz in this and other writings reflects the belief that psychiatric and mental health propaganda have falsely popularized the belief that mental illness is just like any other illness, *when in fact psychiatric and medical problems are fundamentally different.*

To make his point, Szasz described the case of an elderly widow whose husband left the bulk of his $4 million estate to his children, grandchildren, charities, and one-third to his wife. After her husband died, the widow began to give her money away to her widowed sisters, to charities, and finally to distant relatives abroad. After a few years, the children urged her not to waste the money, but the widow continued doing what she felt was right. The children then consulted an attorney in order to have their mother declared mentally incompetent to manage her own affairs. The conflict which followed led the children to seek her commitment in a psychiatric hospital, where she died, and her will leaving the remaining assets to distant relatives was easily broken.

Another example Szasz gave was of a thirty-two-year-old woman who had just delivered her seventh child. Her husband was only sporadically employed and a heavy drinker. Szasz notes that she became depressed after each of her last three babies and had to stay in the hospital a few extra days. During the last confinement she complained of exhaustion and said she ought to die. The woman was overwhelmed by her situation, but could not stay in the hospital without a genuine obstetrical illness. A psychiatrist diagnosed her condition as postpartem depression and committed her to the state mental hospital.

In the first case, Szasz pointed out that the involuntary commitment of persons to mental hospitals by psychiatrists often helps families and society escape from those they find annoying. The purpose, obviously, is not a medical service for the patient but for those whom he or she upsets. In the second case, Szasz reported that the mental hospital provided a patient a medically-approved escape from everyday responsibilities which were too difficult. The escape was not a genuine medical service, but the expression of the only means society has found for dealing with such problems of living.

Szasz's analysis points out these examples as moral and social problems, *not medical problems.* Whether someone is judged sane or insane depends to a certain extent upon the way he affects others, particularly those with whom he is in frequent contact, and also whether or not society has any other means to assist a person.

To summarize, one view holds that abnormal behavior is like any other form of illness. An alternative view treats abnormal behavior as a problem of living similar to other social problems, related to social norms and values, rather than to biological processes. Neither medicine nor psychiatry has developed appropriate concepts to describe abnormality of the psyche as similar to abnormality of the body. A neutral, but descriptively accurate term for mental illness is *behavior disorder*. Behavior disorders can be discussed and viewed from many different levels of explanation—biological, psychological, and social; the framework provided by behavior disorder as a concept is more convenient and general than the restrictive term, mental illness. Indeed, we can expect useful biological concepts to be proposed, but these biological concepts must be viewed in a wider context, such as is implied by behavior disorder, rather than in the narrow concept of illness. Of course one can talk of social ills, but this broadens the term illness to make it meaningless and destroys a useful distinction between social processes and bodily functions. Important practical consequences depend on whether or not this distinction is made, particularly with respect to who is identified as a patient, who may work with them, and the type of training they should have.

A further distinction between illness as a health problem and behavior disorders as a social problem is possible. One can be declared "mentally ill" usually by several mental health experts, or by a legal action in court with a vote of twelve men. In fact, just as a criminal may plead innocent and yet be placed in jail, so may a person plead sanity but be placed in a psychiatric hospital against his will, even if he denies his desire for help and has violated no civil or criminal law. The final appeal in the case of madness is to social norms and the opinion of a mental health expert, not to biological norms. Behavior disorders are a social problem, not a health problem. Let us consider, in detail, commitment to a psychiatric hospital as a new posture for further inspecting the dimensions of madness.

Psychiatric hospitalization

It is important at the outset to realize some of the consequences of being declared mentally ill. At the very least, one's right to vote is lost, the driver's license may be revoked, and the right to make legally binding documents and contracts is voided. It is hard for a former mental patient to reestablish himself in the community, and it is often just as hard to get a job as if he were an ex-convict. Involuntary psychiatric hospitalization has many social consequences, and they are closely related to the issue of civil liberties. A person's constitutional freedoms and rights can be suspended if he is declared mentally ill, and this declaration can be made without due process.[2] Commitment procedures per se will be considered first and then the larger ethical and abstract concepts about how behavior disorders are to be viewed will be considered.

All states have commitment procedures. Some relative or public authority begins the process. Usually two doctors certify to civilian authorities that in their judgment the patient should be placed in a mental hospital. A judge then signs the necessary papers, which commits the patient to the hospital. Dr. H. A. Davidson, a former president of the American Psychiatric Association, writing in the *American Handbook of Psychiatry,* explains that psychiatrists are often impatient with the legal details, and because they view psychosis as a disease it "should no more need formal legal adjudication than does pneumonia or appendicitis."[3]

Davidson goes on to call "infuriating" commitment procedures which would require advance notification to the involuntary patient. His reasoning is that the mad person may flee or be driven to violence or even suicide by such notice. The thrust of his argument is that obsession with legal procedures and the legal rights of the patient fails to protect his medical rights adequately. Davidson points out, however, that there is now a growing legal basis (supported by organized psychiatry) for the thought that, if in psychiatric opinion advanced notification or even appearance in court to challenge the commitment would be harmful to the mental health of the patient, his rights are fully protected by having an attorney receive the notice and appear in the patient's behalf.

In actual practice, and what is favored by the American Psychiatric Association, is a process whereby a physician has power to commit; the standard is the physician's (not necessarily a psychiatrist's) own judgment. This is justified as being in the best interest of the patient. An impartial judge—the physician—can commit a sick person to a psychiatric hospital for treatment, whether or not the patient concurs. In fact, disagreement with the judgment of the mental health agent may be taken as further proof of the mental illness. Further, involuntary commitment can take place behind the scenes—the hearing and the decision being made with the victim unaware of the "charges" against him. But organized psychiatry reacts negatively to the word "charges," for their stated purpose is not to confine people unnecessarily but to help those who need help—whether or not they themselves recognize it.

Suppose that two policemen came to your house to take you to a psychiatric hospital. What can one do? Consider the following illustration. The first thing you learn is that the people you must deal with—the policemen and the minor mental health officials—will not be very communicative. They will not advise you of your legal recourses or discuss in detail the reasons you are being taken to a psychiatric hospital. They will not want to "upset" you. At the hospital, you will probably be told to wait for Dr. So-and-So, who will see you later.

If you wanted to, you could say that the whole proceeding was ridiculous. You could yell and scream, stomp your feet in rage, perhaps start a fist fight, and try to get away. Another person could get a gun, hole up in the attic of his house, and keep the public health officials at bay until they smoked him out with tear gas. But none of these would be a very convincing argument for sanity. The involuntary patient who expects to prove his sanity must go along peaceably with the proceedings and allow himself to be transported quietly to a psychiatric hospital.

Once there, most people will treat the patient condescendingly, for he is assumed to be crazy by virtue of the fact that he is there. He or she might spend an entire day or maybe even longer waiting for the doctor. Given the ratio of several hundred patients for each psychiatrist, psychologist, and social worker in many state psychiatric hospitals, it is physically impossible for the necessary people to see him quickly. In the interim period of one, two, three, or more days while a patient waits, he or she can get no straight answers from anyone. Requests for information will be met by the same standard answer. "Try to relax and wait until the doctor comes." During this period, the patient will stand in line for his meals; sleep in a room without a door with several other people; get up at six or seven in the morning and go to bed at 9:30 at night; urinate and defecate in a toilet stall without a door, and that's about it except for television, reading old magazines, and playing checkers. If the patient becomes agitated, someone will come along and give him a sedative, at the same time noting on his record that the patient needed a sedative. If he refuses the sedative, it might take two or three people to force it down, also duly noted in the record. Commitment gives the hospital all rights for treatment. Finally, when the doctor arrives, the patient might rush up to him, grab him by the collar, shove him against the wall, and bombast him for all that has happened. The patient could then explain that the hospitalization was completely unnecessary, fraudulent, and contrived on the outside by relatives who were unhappy with the way he or she was managing his money or his life. Of course, this kind of behavior is apt to get the patient locked up in a padded cell and told that someone will be back to see him when he quiets down. Again, these happenings will be duly recorded.

Of course, a more peaceful approach may be the most appropriate way out of the involuntary hospitalization, but this requires a long talk with the doctor who will be, at best, only lukewarm about listening to the patient's description of the plots against him. And of course, if the patient was visibly distressed, upset, and somewhat incoherent, all that will be duly noted. The doctor will then ask him some questions that he would probably prefer not to answer: information about his past; his feelings toward different people; how much he drinks; his anxieties; and uncertainties. If he refuses to answer personal questions, he will be regarded as un-cooperative, suspicious, and perhaps paranoid. Whatever he says may be held against him. Whatever he does not say may also be held against him.

If the patient remained sensible and if the hospitalization was manufactured for the convenience of others, it could probably be straightened out, at the expense of no more than two or three weeks of the patient's time plus whatever personal indignities he might have suffered in the hospital and the community at large. If a patient knew his legal right to obtain a writ of *habeas corpus*, bringing suit against the hospital, he could reduce the time considerably. The chances are that educated persons could figure out that they needed to retain an attorney, but if one is poor or uneducated, obtaining a quick discharge would not be so easy.

Nevertheless, even if one knew one's legal rights, they still might not be easy to implement. Some hospitals, as was the practice in a hospital where I worked, read all outgoing mail. The hospital was careful not to tamper with the United States mail. There was simply no mail box on the premises. If a patient wanted a letter mailed, he had to give it *unsealed* to a nurse who would pass it on to the physician, who would read it, mail it for the patient, or return it. A patient could seal a letter, and keep it private, and no one would tamper with it, but it would never reach a mailbox. Of course, there's always the telephone. But the telephone is located on the other side of a locked door. In mental hospitals, it requires permission to use the telephone. It is a pay telephone, so the patient needs a dime. However, all personal possessions and money are taken from patients on admittance and conveniently dropped into an envelope and put in a locked cabinet for safekeeping. Of course, the patient could tell a visitor of his plight and ask someone on the outside to take care of the arrangements for him. This would require that someone on the outside was really interested and knew where the patient was. As a last resort, a patient could go to the barred window and scream at passers-by on the street and plead with someone to come to his aid. He might even fly paper airplane notes to the ground below (provided he could steal some paper and a pencil) starting out "I am trapped in a mental hospital even though I am not crazy," and so forth.

The way out of this nightmarish situation is for an attorney to obtain a writ of *habeas corpus*, thus bringing suit against the hospital superintendent for a hearing before a judge, naming the hospital and the staff as adversaries. It is then incumbent upon the hospital and those seeking commitment to establish in a public hearing that you are crazy and it will permit you to defend yourself against the charges. However, as Szasz notes, this protection is not effective, because most patients do not know how to use it, no effort is made to teach them, and there is no requirement that they be informed.[4] In fact,

Szasz suggests that psychiatrists purposely keep this information from patients.

The important question is not whether *habeas corpus* is a sufficient protection. A psychiatric hospitalization deprives a person of his civil liberties, and *habeas corpus* is the legal safeguard for a person deprived of liberty. The crucial question is whether or not the concept of mental illness and the commitment procedures emerging from this view are appropriate. Part of the problem is to decide which criteria should be used for determining what is appropriate. There is a fine line between protecting a person's civil liberties on the one hand, and providing for a public system of *involuntary* psychiatric hospitalization on the other. Fundamental to a resolution of the interplay between psychiatry and the law is a conception of the nature of madness.

The problem (as long as madness is considered an illness) is how to reconcile the seemingly incompatible needs of protecting civil liberties and providing for involuntary hospitalization. The problem can be solved either by relinquishing our belief in civil liberties, by changing our views of the grounds for providing involuntary hospitalization, or by viewing madness as a behavior disorder rather than illness.

An appropriate solution is one which does not require a loosening or denial of civil liberties, as do the current mental health practices and as did the Inquisition. It will not be until the last chapter before all of the constraints have been considered.

The above example was not intended to imply that "railroading" people into a psychiatric hospital is a frequent occurrence. Notice, however, that the term "false hospitalization" was not used. This is precisely because the problem of what is a "true" or "false" hospitalization is one of the points under discussion, and one that hinges on the fundamental question of the nature of behavior disorders. Clearly, the goal of psychiatry is to make hospitalization a medical and not a legal matter. However, if people can be put in psychiatric hospitals without their consent, we need to examine the basis for this action, since it does have far-reaching social consequences. The problem has been forcefully and dramatically discussed by psychologist Edward Sulzer.[5]

Sulzer compares the mental health expert with the extreme anti-communist and finds both meet the defining characteristics of demagogues. One view assumes there is an international communist conspiracy which must be combated in the name of democracy. The mental health expert assumes many of the problems of our society are due to mental incompetence which must be cured in the name of public health and welfare. Both seek special powers and privileges outside of normal legal restrictions for their mission of labeling others communists or mentally ill. The criteria for this task are so vague that they seek to have their judgments accepted as those of unquestioned expertise. In the field of abnormal psychology and psychiatry, the American Psychological Association and the American Psychiatric Association have successfully sought to establish this special and unquestioned role of mental health expert.

Sulzer made an extreme comparison in his statements about the two professional groups. His charge, however, should not be taken lightly. The implications of the term "mental illness" need to be examined in a wide context and contrasted with various alternatives. The principal alternative for making this contrast is based on behavior, and subsequently will be developed in greater detail. For now, we must remember that the concept of mental illness is strictly an invention, and like other invented ideas it must be evaluated on other grounds so that its usefulness and its limitations can become known.

As might be expected, Szasz has similar views. He too objects to the role of the mental health expert in defining and thereby determining who has mental illness, noting that to continue to see state hospital psychiatrists as people who labor for the mentally ill is to exclude the possibility of change.[6] This conclusion is addressed not to the intentions or motivations of the individuals, but to the system that is supported by the notion of mental illness.

I am not against psychiatric hospitals nor public support of psychiatric hospitals. They serve an important and necessary role in our society. I am against obfuscating and hiding the reasons they exist and I am vehemently opposed to involuntary commitment being hidden behind a concept of illness. This is contrary to our stated concept of an open and free society. It is conceptually backward and is a negative (rather than positive) contribution to the solution of the so-called mental health problem.

The central question is, put simply, how are we to define madness? To see the phenomenon as mental illness and as a medical problem is one alternative; but this implies that it is a health problem and should be left to the experts who profess to know what personality is and how it should be. Psychological processes are to be evaluated and judged in illness-like terms. An alternative view argues that social values and social norms are at stake and that madness is a behavioral disorder and should be evaluated and handled as a social problem. The alternative viewpoint defines a different set of experts, procedures, and criteria for handling the problem. The former view dominates the mental-health movement. The former view looks to the personality, or what we have called the psychodynamic view of the individual, in order to conceptualize mental illness. The alternative view looks more to behavior and to public appraisal of the individual and his problems of living. One stance is an appeal to health standards and the other to social values and circumstances as the broader framework.

Both Sulzer and Szasz favor an open and public approach to the problem of involuntary commitment, but only through full legal processes, rather than by expert judgment. They reject the unquestioned opinion of the mental health expert because he simply is not equipped to make medical decisions about matters of social control. The alternative is to hold people responsible for their own behavior. It is possible to argue that due process should be relaxed in the service of doing something for troubled people. I disagree. But this issue is better left open while we consider further the two alternatives and some of their implications.

7

a
pair
of
alternatives

As was indicated at the conclusion of the last chapter, the mental illness-behavior disorder issue may be seen as parallel to a psychodynamic versus behavioral alternative. But, this is true only to a certain extent.

Now, the psychodynamic and the behavioral alternatives will be examined in their own right. In many ways, these alternatives are broad position labels, representing a general dimension along which many issues fall; issues extending from diagnosis, psychiatry, the law, the nature of psychological theory, the principles of psychotherapy, research strategy, moral philosophy, and social planning.

85

The psychodynamic alternative

The psychodynamic view of abnormal behavior heavily emphasizes past experiences. It views the emergence of personality as a process whereby the social and the emotional experiences of the individual, particularly at an early age, produced the various structural and dynamic aspects the personality will adopt.

The superego is the structural concept in personality which is responsible for one's sense of conscience and guilt, the development of which is assumed to depend upon specific experiences. One extreme is a condition in which the child does not resolve the oedipal conflict, and, instead of developing an identification with his father and internalizing parental values (the development of conscience), he develops a hatred of his father, does not identify, and therefore does not develop a conscience. The result in terms of personality, engendered by an unloving, punitive father, is the affectionless psychopath who can cause others pain without guilt and perhaps with pleasure, because he is really punishing society (the father) for its unloving treatment of him. The psychopath's difficulty is a defective psychological structure (the superego) stemming from a disturbance in the affective nature of the father-son relationship. [1]

All the significant aspects of personality, from a psychodynamic point of view, are related to such early childhood experiences. The crucial factor in understanding madness is identifying those ingredients of a personality that are distorted, out of balance, or which represent unhealthy compensations. The task of treatment is to rectify the defective structure or process within the personality. The change aims at a reconstruction of the personality, for that is the fundamental source of the difficulty.

AN ILLUSTRATION. An excellent delineation of the logic of this viewpoint is provided in a book entitled *Dialogues with Mothers* by Bruno Bettelheim. In a section entitled "The Potty and the Piggy Bank," Bettelheim provides the transcript of a discussion with a group of mothers.[2] One mother presented the problem of her three-year-old daughter who wet her pants. The mother reported she hadn't been concerned about it until the grandparents visited and found it terrible that she was not toilet-trained. The frequency of her child's wetting got worse and the mother felt that something needed to be done, especially since she had all that extra diaper washing to do. Since the child was dry at nursery school and only wet at home, the discussion focused on why. Various reasons were suggested, e.g., the child was making extra work for the mother as revenge and would stop wetting if the mother sent the diapers out and didn't seem so concerned about them. To the suggestion that she ignore the problem, the mother said she had put up with two kittens and their puddles and could probably put up with her daughter's.

At this point, Bettelheim inquired about when the kittens were obtained and their sex. They were ex-males. When Dr. Bettelheim inquired whether the child knew that, the mother explained no, that the child didn't know enough about such things to find out or to inquire. He then stated he was against castrating pets because children will be afraid someone will do that to them. He proposed that children at that age start to look for sex differences, and at nursery school the children are often interested in watching others in the toilet. Once they notice sex differences, they begin looking for them, and if something is missing, the children will wonder who is responsible, because young children identify so much with animals.

At this point, another member of the group

remembered that the same mother had spoken once of the time her little girl had put one of the cats on the toilet as if it were a child. The cat fell in and naturally the mother had to pull it out. Bettelheim suggested that the child had a vivid memory of what had happened to the cat. He also mentioned the fact that the girl might believe that the nursery school toilet was safe because no kitten had fallen into it. The discussion was concluded by Bettelheim, who said the castration of the cats may have been the important factor, or the disapproval of the grandparents, or the cat nearly drowning, or all three. The group session had helped the mother discover the facts involved and she knew it was up to her to use the information and to try out one approach after another until something worked.

At the next meeting, two weeks later, the mother was asked about the cats. She said they had decided not to give the cats away because she didn't believe castrated cats caused complexes and because the wetting problem was solved. She and her husband at first had tried to show their daughter that they weren't really upset about her wetting but the mother confessed that they were actually fuming underneath. At this point, they simply told the child that they didn't like her wetting and to please stop. They got down the old potty chair so that the girl didn't have to use the potty seat on the large toilet. At the same time, the little girl found a great big piggy bank and discovered that pennies would disappear into it and rattle around. The mother put the piggy bank beside the potty chair and told her daughter that if she used the potty before she got her pants wet they would give her pennies to put into the slot. It worked.

But Bettelheim was not impressed. He pointed out that spanking works too, but what the parents had done was even worse, that it was psychologically unsound, and could upset the girl's life. The parents, he explained, had established a connection between money and elimination. The incident was included in his book as a lesson on how compulsive symptoms come into being. The girl, when forced to let go of body content in the toilet, would hold onto money instead.

The foregoing example illustrates many of the prevalent notions in clinical and psychiatric theory today. A few aspects of the case should be examined in order to illustrate the reliance of psychodynamic theory on invented structures and processes.

The castrated cat, for example, and the concern over elimination illustrate the prominence given to these areas as the basis for subsequent personality development. The castration is important, because if the cat had lost something and if the mother had caused it, maybe she is also responsible for the child missing something. Presumably, the resentment or fear over being deprived of an outward genital by the parents could be responsible, in the short run, for the girl's resisting toilet training, and in the long run might conceivably result in an over-concern with the genitalia. Such concern could result in the girl's failure to identify with the mother who deprived her of a penis and could result in a long-lasting resentment against women in general and femininity in particular. Under these conditions, we can imagine the girl spending the rest of her life seeking symbolically to replace the penis deprived her by her mother. After all, she was presumably wetting while standing up, just as if she did have a penis.

Of course, many adults find this kind of logic irrational, but it is defended as being close to a child's level of reasoning at age three and all such experience has its psychological impact on the personality of the child. The personality (not the logic) stays with her and will determine how she reacts in future situations.

But the central point is reflected in Dr. Bettelheim's two angry rebukes of the mother: "If you want to make your child. . .what is described in books as an anal erotic, go ahead and do that." And, ". . .but you have established a connection between money and elimination which never existed before in her mind. . .you have established a connection between two such terribly important things in our society: money and cleanliness."

The psychodynamic theorist sees the personality being shaped by such significant experiences as these. Cleanliness and bodily elimination become a source of pleasure and value; personal worth and the value society places on money could be achieved through cleanliness. The dangerous outcome feared by Bettelheim is an adult who strives for these values and for self-respect through obsessive concern with cleanliness and neatness. Bodily elimination becomes a fixation—an area of intense preoccupation—a source of pleasure and security at the expense of other aspects of living.

Of course, we will probably never know the actual outcome of this girl's experience. It is unlikely that one such experience could have such far-reaching effects, but the accumulation of such events is assumed to be irreversible in personality development. The use of the potty chair won parental approval. If the mother is—as she was painted—a person who values dryness more than the ingenuity of her child, then the stage is set for the further purchase of self-regard through cleanliness.

Many examples could have been selected for this section. The purpose is to highlight the complex interplay between social-emotional experiences, the resulting personality structure, and the long-term effort to live in the real world. The effectiveness of the personality depends in part on its flexibility in adapting to the demands made by the environment. The hypothetical adult woman extrapolated from the Bettelheim example could perhaps find a satisfying, useful existence working in the sanitary interior of a surgical room and living an old maid's existence in a house never muddied by children's feet. But she would·be taxed, perhaps beyond the breaking point, by the demands of being wife to a man who sweated profusely and squeezed his toothpaste from the middle of the tube, or mother to a child with colitis.

The behavioral alternative

The psychodynamic and behavioral alternatives share certain similarities, but on another level, they are so different that one wonders if they really are comparable at all. The similarity is the assumption of a psychological cause that both share. Like the psychodynamic, the behavioral alternative assumes the behavior of the organism is acquired over its life history. The unique experiences determine the nature of the organism.

The difference is to be seen in how the effects of these previous experiences are to be conceptualized. The behavioral alternative does not try to infer the particular events that have led up to a particular behavior. It does not attempt to invent a personality or self to sit between those earlier socializing events and the behavioral characteristics of the individual. It merely looks at the behavior. The behavior itself and what perpetuates it are the only explanation that is needed.

AN ILLUSTRATION. As a contrast to Bettelheim's reaction to the way the mother toilet-trained a three-year-old girl by using money, we will now look at what was recommended in a case report by Charles Madsen, a behavioral psychologist.[3] He hypothesized that toilet training could be made more rapid and less stressful if the principles of learning were used. A child's mother consulted Madsen as to the best method to train her nineteen-month-old girl in the shortest possible time because the family was planning an extended automobile trip within a month.

Madsen first determined that there was

91

probably physiological readiness, evidenced by the fact that the child had remained dry on a number of occasions at both nap and bedtime. The mother had purchased a small toilet and allowed the child to sit on it whenever she wanted to. Also about four times a day the mother had placed the child on the toilet and stayed with her. At the time of consultation, there had been no successful eliminations and the child was beginning to cry and react negatively to being placed on the toilet.

Madsen suggested the child be offered a candy reward for a successful elimination. After a dry diaper in the morning or after a nap, the child was placed on the potty and read to or otherwise entertained. She was allowed to leave the toilet at anytime. At each placement, she was told she would receive candy if she "went" on the toilet. The second placement resulted in a success. She received her candy, was praised, and told she would get candy each time she used the toilet. On the fourth day, the child said "urinate a toto, get candy," and on the fifth day the child was allowed to ask to be taken to the toilet instead of being placed on the toilet after a dry diaper. By the twelfth day the child was trained. After the fifteenth day, the candy was given only if requested. The automobile trip occurred without an accident and sixty days after the start of the program, the request for candy was zero and the child was using the bathroom on her own.

Madsen suggested that such a training program has many positive advantages. The conflict between mother and child, already starting to appear before she consulted the psychologist, was eliminated, there was rapid training in a way which was comfortable for the mother and for the child, and self-control was fostered through the capability to act successfully. Madsen further reported that after four and one-half years, there had been no unpleasant consequences, and the child has developed normally.

The first and most striking feature of this illustration is the simple, straightforward view of human behavior. Implicit in the handling of the case is the belief that much of what we are is what we do, and what we do depends on what responses are learned and maintained. Responses which produce desirable outcomes and avoid unpleasant ones are learned. When the rewards are given only under certain conditions, such as using the toilet, a discrimination is made; then the one response becomes frequent, and the other response is eventually forgotten. The candy was incidental, except that it was effective as motivation for the child's cooperation at the time of training. Once the execution of the response was mastered, the withdrawal of the candy was inconsequential, since other positive reinforcement, parental praise and approval, maintained the desired toilet habits. From this view, talk about effects on personality having long-term consequences for a wide range of human activities (tolerance of sweaty men, the type of leisure activities that would be enjoyed, etc.) is little short of ridiculous.

Commentary

In choosing the use of the toilet as my example, I have deliberately used what may seem like an extremely simple or perhaps trivial comparison. But I don't think it is. Bettelheim was concerned about the girl becoming an anal-erotic woman. Madsen was concerned about the girl learning to use the toilet. This difference, regardless of simplicity, illustrates an important, basic difference in the ways of viewing man.

Of course, many aspects of human behavior are more complex than learning to use the toilet. But so too are behavioral theories of social learning and motivation more complex than caramel candy. These theories have been developed over time in experimental psychology by studying a variety of animals—rats, dogs, monkeys, and man—performing a variety of tasks. The outcome of the research is a serious attempt to use the general process of learning and motivation to understand how complex human social responses and discriminations are acquired, maintained, and changed. The complexity and the social nature of the circumstances make some types of inquiry difficult, *but the basic assumption is that personality consists of the things a person has learned to do or not to do.*

By proposing a behavioral alternative, we have obviously not changed man's nature or even the kinds of behavior we wish to understand. We have changed the conceptual inventions used to achieve our ends. Although arbitrary, the decisions about the best ways of viewing events are not to be made lightly. These decisions require a further examination of the subject matter from different perspectives.

Dynamic-behavioral alternatives

It should be emphasized that the two case studies about toilet training prove nothing. They only illustrate different conceptual approaches. We can, however, infer something about Bettelheim's and Madsen's views of human behavior. These views are our primary concern (not the details of a dynamic or a behavioral recommendation for toilet-training or sundry child-rearing problems). The major issue is the nature of the conceptual system used.

What we see in these examples are two radically different approaches to human behavior. The dynamic is more molar and holistic, and the behavioral more molecular and specific. The dynamic uses concepts of psychological states and processes, whereas the behavioral uses concepts based on the operations which influence the occurrence of actions. The psychodynamic concepts are considered by the behaviorists as being unscientific, untestable, and therefore inadequate as "science." On the other hand, the behavioral concepts are seen by dynamicists as being trivial, incomplete, and an attempt to handle complex human behavior with ideas that are only appropriate for the white rat.

To a certain extent, these differences rest in beliefs, not facts. The behavioral alternative chooses to build slowly upon existing concepts and work toward the complex; the dynamic chooses to work with the whole, insisting that a person can be understood only as an entire entity. There are no answers to these questions, but the issue refers in part to fundamental differences of opinion about the appropriate procedures for coming to understand, predict, and control behavior.

The division between a psychodynamic and behavioral alternative parallels some of the perspectives presented previously. Consider first the problem of diagnosis. What is to be diagnosed? The psychodynamic view tends to be correlated with an illness approach. It implies an optimal, or at least an adjusted, personality system with the various components working together in harmony. Mental illness is a breakdown within this system. A specific form of mental illness depends on what systems are functioning improperly. From this view, the advancement of knowledge about mental illness involves, in part, understanding the particular personal systems and mechanisms that are functioning improperly, and in part, developing more precise, useful conceptualizations of the various personality systems, mechanisms, and their interrelationships. The use of these terms implies psychological systems that are similar to organ systems. Health or illness represents the functioning level of these systems, implying that psychological systems can be evaluated (diagnosed) just as the functioning of many organ systems can now be tested, X-rayed, or otherwise assessed.

As an illustration, consider the answer given by Dr. Daniel Blain, former president of the American Psychiatric Association, in an interview.[4] To a question about a periodic mental health check-up, Blain gave an unqualified yes. A mental check-up was suggested for people who are "psychologically vulnerable," such as children entering puberty, persons about to marry or change jobs, men in their early forties, and older people. Who is left?

The mental health posters have not yet advertised an annual or biannual check-up as is recommended for affluent people's teeth. But the sound of mental health is in the air. We are on the verge of being urged to scrub and deodorize our personalities and publicly display good mental health. Psychological exercises to strengthen one's character are a not too distant or too far-fetched extension of this trend. The ultimate implication is an absolute view of the nature of normality.

By contrast, the behavioral alternative is to move away from an illness notion toward a behavioral-disorder or problems-of-living approach. Here the emphasis is on the person's actions. Nonobservable psychological processes, systems, mechanisms, and their intricate balance are rendered relatively unimportant, and in some extremes, are ignored completely. Rather, various responses made in different situations result in certain consequences. The individual's behavior cannot be judged as healthy or sick, in the sense of an absolute psychological evaluation. This is a learned behavior having outcomes more or less satisfactory to someone—the patient, the child's parents, society in general, or even the therapist. An evaluation must, in any case, be based on some notion, or someone's notion, *of how the person should behave.*

Establishing a list of acceptable and unacceptable behaviors is no small task. Such a task, of course, introduces some new and different problems of ethics and social values than those involved in the dynamic or total personality approach.

The two approaches to abnormal psychology may also be compared with respect to considerations of civil liberties and involuntary commitment. The dynamic approach makes its recommendations in terms of personality processes. An individual may be deprived by society of his civil liberties or excused from responsibility for a crime committed because of what he is as a person (his characteristics and traits). Whereas, from a behavioral alternative, an individual may be deprived of civil liberties for what he does (his behavior) and, if we take Szasz as our example, treated as if he were responsible for his behavior. Thus, public and open criteria must be used as guides for actions, as contrasted to the advice of a mental health expert, who examines the overall personality of the individual in question.

How is one to decide between the various issues and problems? It would seem wise to give this evaluation dilemma some serious thought now, so that it may be kept in mind before going any further.

It is impossible to avoid making some judgment about the alternative views of abnormal behavior. The option of waiting to see how it all turns out is both unacceptable and impossible for several reasons: (1) Decisions about individual people must be made daily, and implicit in any decision is an option for one perspective or another. The necessity for making decisions will not go away. At the first line of responsibility these decisions involve the psychological and psychiatric professions, but they also involve the taxpayer and the individual who must live with the social and ethical values implicit in the decisions and options that are made. (2) There must be some criteria from which to make a judgment between the alternatives when there are critical encounters. But an agreement between the proponents of the two alternatives presents a problem in itself. The grounds used to define a critical encounter are also relative and depend on assumptions made at other levels. It is only through a constant search for such criteria that progress results. And (3), most important, is the necessity for intellectual commitment and open-mindedness. Only through continual evaluation can one insure that a particular viewpoint does not become a "religion" with its dogma accepted on faith. Open-mindedness exists only when alternatives and implicit assumptions are examined at all levels. Open-minded evaluation in which the shortcomings of one's own approach are seen as clearly as its accomplishments assures a commitment to action based on assumptions and social values which are explicit and acceptable on rational grounds, given the here and now, but forward-looking toward newer ideas.

An important aspect of behavior disorders is the fact that there are over 700,000 hospitalized persons and uncounted numbers of outpatients. The problem will not go away—although it can be made larger or smaller by the definition of madness. One of the tasks is to examine the social values and scientific status of the concepts that must be used to set the boundaries for a definition of a behavior disorder and a prescription for action. The conditions under which psychopathology may be said to exist, the type of decisions to be made, and the inescapable demands on the psychological and psychiatric professions are part of the reality of the situation. This reality adds a further dimension that has not yet received sufficient attention in this book. So far we have dealt with *abstract* considerations which oversimplify considerably the nature of the problem. But to act as if these abstractions were the only considerations is to make a judgment that those who are responsible for patients are not willing to grant. A new dimension can be added by considering the work-a-day encounters between persons who are considered mad and the mental health profession.

8

clinical
formulations

A practicing clinical psychologist or psychiatrist is frequently called upon to make decisions that can have far-reaching effects on other people's lives. The decision, for example, to hospitalize a mother affects the patient, her husband, and their children. Other decisions, such as the decision to confine a person to a psychiatric hospital, perhaps against his or her wishes, have both legal and social consequences. With respect to criminal law, a psychiatric decision may determine whether a person goes to jail or is placed in a psychiatric hospital. In this chapter we will consider first the clinical decisions a therapist makes in the daily treatment and management of his patients. And, in the next chapter, the validity and the accuracy of the decisions themselves and the process whereby they are reached.

Some general considerations

When a clinician is called upon to make such far-reaching decisions about his patients, he usually does so on the basis of his clinical formulation of the patient and the situation. A clinical formulation is a more or less explicitly worked-out set of expectations about what will happen given one decision or another on his part. The formulation must include some beliefs about the patient's personality, the nature of his or her circumstances, and how they combine. It is a form of explanation which yields predictions about outcomes and therefore provides a basis for the decision.

For example, assume that a patient who is given to self-blame has made some progress. If the therapist does not give him or her a weekend pass, these individuals may become discouraged about the lack of progress and become depressed. But if the therapist does send a patient home for a visit and things go poorly, the progress made to date in building confidence may be destroyed. On the other hand, a good visit could help the treatment process.

Since it is impossible to know with certainty what a patient will in fact do, one must consider and evaluate the range of situations and outcomes that might occur. On the basis of these anticipated outcomes, such as building or destroying confidence, and their likelihood of occurrence, the decision must be made. A clinical formulation of *some form*—no matter how simple-minded or intuitive—must precede any clinical decision. Assumptions about human behavior and a guess as to what behavior will occur are at least implicit, if not explicit, in a decision. Once an explicit formulation of a patient is put together it then may be used for anticipating the patient's behavior in numerous other situations.

Because there are many inferences to be made before a decision is reached, the possibility exists of making errors. An improper formulation is likely, of course, to lead to a poor decision, or if it leads to a good decision, it is for the wrong reasons. Errors may occur because the formulations or the environmental situations that the patient must deal with were incorrectly evaluated or because the process of how the patient's personality and the anticipated environmental situations interact could not be solved as could an equation. It is often difficult to evaluate the clinical formulation and decision-making process simply because it is difficult to know just exactly what can be concluded. The problem of evaluating clinical formulations has not been solved, either in abstract or practical terms.

We need to be able to evaluate the decision-making process in order to learn from mistakes and to improve the theory. We need to tear apart the rules for making decisions and prognoses, for evaluating the patient's environment, and for making predictions of behavior. But the nature of the problem and the practical circumstances have made such information difficult to get for several reasons:

INVARIANCE. There is a large amount of *variance* in people's behavior and in the multitude of situations they encounter. Put simply, people are different and every clinical diagnosis has some unique aspects that set it apart from experiences of other people. The same may be said of situations; no two are identical. Yet, predictions are based on an assumption of invariance. The clinician must assume for *practical purposes*, that if a patient is of such-and-such a type, if the situation has this and that characteristic, then x is likely to happen. We can see here the use of an "if this, then that" type of reasoning. The relevant dimensions must be attended to and the irrelevant dimensions—which help to make the situation unique—ignored. An arbitrary preemptive decision must be made, as when a therapist determines self-blame to be the central issue and when some other issue, such as headaches, is considered irrelevant or secondary.

When a prediction based on such judgments is not supported, there is no way to do it over again in order to try something else. Unfortunately, one must wait until a similar situation occurs and then try other alternatives; but, the next situation is not a replication of the previous person and his situation and unbiased conclusions are not possible. Of course, this is true of any empirical test, but the information contributed by a "replication" varies widely according to the fidelity with which a condition can be repeated for further evaluation. To reproduce any given number of pounds of air pressure is relatively free of significant time-to-time variation. The replication of the intensity of hunger by manipulating hours of deprivation of food has less fidelity than pounds of air, but is still high. However, the type of situations the clinician is faced with is not convincingly invariant, i.e., replications are hard to come by.

The development of rules requires a broad sample of the persons and situations in various relevant dimensions in order to establish the "if this, then that" relationship. Hard and fast rules do not exist partly because there are still no sound concepts to identify the significant variations. This is, in turn, difficult because the concepts themselves cannot be evaluated without ambiguity.

The applied clinical situation is not a happy one for obtaining data or for verifying the process being used. Situations can seldom, if ever, be contrived as they are in laboratory experiments, and frequently the verification process must go on after the fact, using clinicians' memories of what was attended to and what was ignored in relatively unique and complicated situations.

CONSTRUCTS. People and situations can be evaluated only as accurately as our words and ideas permit. We must invent the names and concepts which describe the emotional states and the types of circumstances in which people find themselves. The concepts must accurately reflect the salient and significant aspects of the behavior in question if suitable accuracy of prediction is to be achieved. The concepts we have are gross and inadequate and, due to the lack of invariance, evaluations and refinement are hard to come by. From a scientific standpoint, our current clinical concepts are but a shade better than devils for achieving our ends.

VERIFICATION. The verification task is not logically impossible or even hopeless, it is just difficult. Apart from the lack of invariance and good constructs, there are other practical problems of verification. The person in a position to make clinical decisions is typically not the person who is interested in doing research. The clinician in a state hospital in the course of a day makes numerous decisions; if he has 300 or more patients to care for, he has more than eight hours' work merely to deal hurriedly with pressing physical (medical) and psychological decisions without ever trying to verify them. He is applying rules of thumb to make decisions that must be made. To verify what he is doing would require a great deal of time, thought, and planning; it would require resources which do not exist. The decisions must be made anyway, some of a limited number of dollars must be spent for food and heat, resources are consumed, and the system goes on because it must.

There are psychologists and psychiatrists who are actively engaged in research, but these people also have other duties which make demands on their time. Many research people do not have contact with the patient population in the sense of responsibility for the work-a-day decisions. The pure scientist lives in a world of his own, and the abstractions he works with are often far removed from the needs of the practicing clinician. The study of massed versus distributed practice of learning a list of three-letter nonsense syllables, or of the salivary responses of dogs, must sometimes seem nothing short of trivial to the ward administrator of 500 patients.

Again we come face-to-face with the manpower shortage discussed earlier and with the conclusion of the final report of the Joint Commission recommending the need for more verifiable information and the need to counteract the shortage of trained manpower and inadequate physical facilities. The social realities of the profession are such that no large-scale changes will be made soon. Clinical decisions must provide the ultimate proving grounds for invented abstractions. These proving grounds, however, are not now the focal points for new data or for verification; instead, they perpetuate the application of concepts and procedures the scientist questions as lacking the necessary verification.

EXPLICITNESS. Any decision about treatment for a disturbed patient involves many assumptions about man, madness, and social values. Assumptions are implicit in making any formulation and arriving at any decision. Frequently, however, these assumptions remain implicit as the clinician calls upon his past experience and hurries from one decision to the next. It is only when we can be explicit about the assumptions used in a formulation that it is possible to proceed with the scientific task of concept evaluation. Likewise, it is only when the scientist can provide explicit concepts which the clinician can use unambiguously that he can help test the concepts in actual practice. It is a two-way street, and the vagueness of what is actually done and why, plus the abstract nature of the concepts of the pure scientist, assures that each is virtually useless to the other.

Clinical formulations

Missing from illustrative case histories presented in most textbooks is an examination of the
process of clinical formulations and decisions in a
way which directs attention toward the assumptions
and the general problems involved—problems such
as invariance, constructs, verification, and explicitness. The purpose of the case histories which follow
is to focus on what is currently done and on the
confidence we may have in the reasons for doing it.
The intent of this chapter is not to attack critically
formulations and decisions, but to present an appraisal of the problem of reconciling practical
demands with scientific demands. The two are not
always congenial. It is important not to ignore the
conflicting demands either by presenting an over
glamorized view of the capability of the current
practicing clinician, or by acting from a scientific
posture as if madness were only an abstraction. In
one sense, madness exists more in its practical
implications than as an abstract theoretical concept,
for it is only through the perspective of its day-to-day
management that the ultimate evaluation of the
abstract issues—such as the dynamic-behavioral
alternatives—can be achieved.

Some clinical illustrations

THE HATCHET. The first case involves a woman
who voluntarily signed herself into a psychiatric
hospital. As a voluntary patient, she could not be
kept in the hospital against her wishes longer than
five days after requesting her release. The required
five-day notice which accompanied voluntary admission allowed the hospital to have time to obtain
formal commitment if the authorities felt it was
unwise to allow a voluntary patient to return to the
community.

The patient had heaved a hatchet at her
husband. The hatchet stuck in the wall, missing his

head by a fraction of an inch, but only because he ducked in time. The husband reported that his wife had been acting strangely, and the hatchet incident convinced him she needed psychiatric help. The wife voluntarily signed herself into the hospital, although only after she realized that her husband would have had her committed if she did not go voluntarily. The husband had not pressed assault charges against her and there was no involvement with the police or courts at the time of hospitalization.

In the hospital, the woman very quickly covered over any gross signs of psychopathology. She admitted she had been mixed up, but soon reported that she was well and that the hospital had done her a world of good. She declared she was ready to return to her husband and children and she asked to be released. The husband wanted his wife home, providing she was well again. But he was also prepared, for his own protection, to keep her hospitalized if the doctors thought it was necessary and recommended commitment. Commitment would have been very easy to obtain in this case since it involved a violent, dangerous act. A decision had to be made: obtain commitment and involuntary hospitalization or release the patient? If the woman was released from the hospital, she would return to her home and would be sleeping in the same bed with her husband. If she wanted to make sure she did not miss the second time, she would have ample opportunity. Needless to say, the husband was somewhat concerned about whether or not his wife was well again. So, too, were the hospital authorities.

They felt they had not done anything for the patient. She had gotten too well too fast; she was reluctant to continue psychiatric treatment, maintaining that everything was fine now. At least on the surface, everything was fine. She seemed perfectly congenial, she gave no evidence of gross psychopathology, and she had no traditional symptoms. The woman was evaluated by several psychiatrists and myself. As a clinical psychologist, I administered a battery of psychological tests. Together we sat down to make a decision.

Such decisions are made many times each day, and as is obvious, they are very important decisions, for they involve not only the welfare of the patient, but the welfare of those around the patient. Decisions cannot be taken lightly, yet too often they must be made quickly by an overworked staff. As a participating member of the group, I supported the release of the patient. My decision, along with the others, was based on our formulation of her personality and our expectation of how well she could handle her future encounters with her environment, and the likely outcome of those encounters. We had to weigh the possible alternatives with their possible consequences. On the one hand, a husband and children were in need of a wife and mother. On the other hand, there was their well-being and safety to consider. From the standpoint of the patient, there was the advantage of being able to return to a normal life, to the community, and to fulfill her responsibilities to her family, versus the possibility of a prolonged hospitalization carried out against her wishes with the possibility she would rebel against treatment and perhaps grow bitter toward both the hospital and her husband. Perhaps the hospitalization would be a life-long imprisonment which would have in fact been unnecessary if we had discharged her. But perhaps to discharge her would put a temptation before her that she would not be able to resist and that would lead to murder.

We released her.

I can report that in the two or three months after discharge, while I was still working at the hospital, there were no bad consequences of our decision. However, several months is a very short time and yields incomplete data on which to base a judgment that our evaluation was accurate and best for everyone concerned. I have since left the area, and I have no way of knowing what happened three months, or a year, or even five years later. I have not read in the newspapers of a hatchet murder in the city where they lived, but that is not proof my decision was correct. Perhaps an error was made that I will never know about; although, in my own mind, I am likely to have confirmed the logic used in arriving at the formulation and the inferences I made in coming to my decision. Clearly, without follow-up information these are moot questions that will never have a chance to be considered. Lack of feedback is typical of most clinical formulations and clinical decisions. It is a severe handicap to a critical examination of one's thinking and concepts. It is a problem that hangs heavy over the practical work-a-day necessity of formulation and decision.

Even if the outcome could be determined today, we would have no way of knowing how good the concepts were, and if the decision was wrong, why it was wrong. Was it in the formulation? Was it in an improper evaluation of the situation? Was it faulty logic or deduction? Was it in the reasoning or was it in the nature of the theory used? How could alternative formulations be tested to assess their usefulness?

I have never had to make a similar decision, or even one that was close enough to feel that my experience in the hatchet case helped me. I cannot turn back the hands of time and make a different decision to see what would have happened. But, neither is it clear how this experience should be pooled with others to test concepts or develop rules of thumb. Each decision seems so unique and so different that the lack of invariance from which concepts are built and tested is the striking feature. We are left with man's requirement that man be judged by man, rather than, say, by a flip of a coin:

Heads. Do not discharge! We proceed on the clinician's assumptions about how people work and what madness is, without the means to verify the adequacy of what we do in a way acceptable to even minimum scientific standards. Information about outcomes is rarely available, and always hard to interpret. We rely on what "I remember happening to me" and what others remember happening to them through *illustrative case studies*.

The proof of witchcraft recounted in *Malleus Maleficarum* is built, in part, upon the selectively remembered case studies reported by *reputable* inquisitors. The selective case history is of no more value in verifying current concepts of mental illness than it was in 1487 in verifying the work of the devil.

THE DEPRESSED LADY. I can recall another situation in which I gave a patient psychological tests and later participated in a decision. The therapist presented his case to a staff conference in order to get help on a difficult decision. The question was whether or not to discharge a depressed patient. The therapist felt the woman had a better chance for recovery outside the hospital. He felt that if she remained in the hospital, her depression would probably stabilize, and she would soon settle into the routine of the hospital and become an established chronic patient. He felt all that could be achieved by hospitalization had been achieved, and if this patient was ever to get better, now was the time to capitalize on the improvement that had taken place by getting her back into the community. The prospect for recovery was not good, but perhaps better than waiting with the anticipation of a chronic custodial patient. However, one is always hesitant about discharging a depressed patient, for the danger of suicide is ever present. The case conference considered the case in as much detail *as time permitted*. Various people offered their opinions and reasons for them. I agreed with the

111

therapist that the patient would be better off outside the hospital. Shortly after the meeting, the patient, therapist, and social worker made plans for the discharge which occurred a few days later. In less that twenty-four hours after discharge, the patient made a successful suicide.

This, of course, was one mistake that could not be corrected. Was our formulation of the patient incorrect? Was our assessment of the situation wrong? Or, perhaps, was it by and large a good decision and just a very unlikely chance that the suicide actually occurred? Suppose we knew there was one chance in a hundred that she would commit suicide if she was discharged, but one chance in two she would become a chronic hospitalized patient for the rest of her life if she was not discharged. One choice results in the finality of death, the other in an institutionalized life. What choice do you make? There are other possibilities, of course, but this illustrates the kind of crucial clinical decisions which must be made. They are by no means cut and dried. They are decisions that can never be made lightly and, as this case illustrates, they cannot be made with certainty. But often they must be made quickly. If too much time was spent on the depressed lady and others, the five-day holding period on the hatchet case would have expired with no decision or with the administrator meeting the husband in the lobby and with a flip of a coin saying, "Take her with you."

Seldom is unambiguous feedback available. No two cases are sufficiently similar to provide the 10,000 or so instances necessary to arrive at the figure of one chance in one hundred of suicide, or one in two of becoming a chronic patient. And, even if we did find 10,000 instances to put together, it only would be by means of classification with concepts which are arbitrary themselves and in dire need of verification and refinement. These problems are soluble; but not quickly, especially given the current

112

practical work-a-day situation and the structure of the mental health movement.

The most important observation is that the necessity for making decisions will not go away. We simply cannot start all over again. This is the practical aspect of madness, and the practicing psychiatrist must face it daily. It is the psychodynamic, not the behavioral approach, which provides him with his tools. Hatchet-throwing and suicide are not responses which can be worked with. There is nothing in the behavior that tells the clinician to discharge or not—it is only a clinical formulation, of some sort, which gives him some basis for what he does. The academic psychologist or research psychiatrist can question the verifiability of the dynamic concepts the clinician used, and he can speak in favor of laboratory-based concepts, but he has offered no day-to-day practical alternatives. A moratorium on problems in living is not a feasible or possible alternative. Thus, the decision about what type of concepts to use, what stand to take on diagnoses and so on, throughout the list of topics considered so far, is only in part an academic problem and in part a practical problem.

SELF-RELIANCE. A final illustration concerns the fourth hospitalization of Mrs. C, a twenty-two-year-old married woman with two children. In previous hospitalizations, she had been diagnosed as schizophrenic and on two different occasions received electro-convulsive shock therapy. On the fourth hospitalization, she was diagnosed as having a neurotic disorder with anxiety reaction. This was a questionable diagnosis because the patient was more severely disturbed than the typical anxiety neurotic; some staff members felt she lacked the strength typically associated with neurotic disorders and showed personality weakness more typical of a psychotic disorder, such as schizophrenia. There was disagreement among the staff with the therapist's decision to provide psychodynamic psychotherapy aimed toward a reconstruction of the personality.

The patient had many problems. One of the repetitive themes of her life was failure to take responsibility for her own behavior. Whenever faced with a difficult situation, she would pursue a line of action that was certain to lead to an unhappy outcome. She would thus force someone else to stop her and to make her do what was best. She would fight the person who took responsibility for her every inch of the way—as if to test them. She always made sure that such a person was around and she held on to only those relationships where the other person would do what was best for her, no matter how hard she fought him. She had never taken responsibility for herself; it was someone else's task, and a thankless one, because Mrs. C. continually tested those persons.

One of the patient's assets in life was her husband, who was both tolerant and sympathetic toward her, and in spite of a long, difficult relationship with her, was still able to maintain his interest in her welfare, even though she did not reciprocate his concern. He did what he thought was best for her and suffered the attendant abuse with remarkable tolerance.

As therapy progressed, the patient gained more and more confidence in herself to the point where she was given ground privileges, which permitted her to come and go as she wanted as long as she stayed within certain boundaries and met her scheduled events. She had responsibility for managing her affairs on a miniature scale.

At about this time, she struck up an acquaintance with a male patient who was in the hospital on a voluntary basis. The male patient left the hospital against medical advice, which means that after giving five days' notice, he was released without commitment proceedings. After he left the hospital, Mrs. C. continued to see him by making use of her ground privileges, contrary to the hospital rules. It was against her moral standards to carry on an affair, and not to be overlooked was the fact an affair might jeopardize her relationship with her husband, one of her few assets.

Mrs. C. saw her boyfriend openly, observed on one occasion by a nurse, and on another occasion by a patient with a notorious reputation for betraying trust. As soon as the indirect reports of her activities were called to the attention of the therapist, he confronted the patient with the reports, and she confirmed their accuracy. Mrs. C. said the last time she met her male friend they had taken a car ride and had almost ended up at a motel. She said she didn't know if she could control herself the next time. The therapist asked her if she wanted to be taken off hospital privileges, and she said no, she would only try to leave the hospital if she was restricted. She said she knew what she was doing was against the hospital rules and her own standards, but yet she was going to continue to see him.

The therapist had a clinical formulation of the patient. It was implied by the interpretive comments surrounding the description of the repetitive theme in her life—avoiding responsibility. The formulation (an invention) gave meaning to a series of events in her life. To the therapist, the current incident sounded like a familiar repetition of the old theme. Specifically, in his view, Mrs. C. was forcing him to make a decision for her by acting in a way that was detrimental to her best interest. Her action was intended to reconfirm for herself that the therapist was concerned about her, and would relieve her of the responsibility for the decision to give up the affair. Mrs. C. was able to give a point-by-point account of the ways in which this incident was like countless others in her past and like other encounters between her and the therapist.

The therapist then made a decision to act on the basis of his formulation and his expectations of what the outcome would be. He felt she did not have genuine feelings towards the boyfriend but that he was a convenient object for another neurotic effort to avoid assuming personal responsibility and to reject the demands made upon her when she was given ground privileges. He felt the patient was now strong enough to make her own decision and that the situation would provide an opportunity for personality growth and self-development. He felt that she could and would assume responsibility for her actions and subsequently grow in self-assurance and self-respect.

The therapist pointed out that she had taken great pains to get caught and that she had acknowledged that her actions were wrong for her. He commented that she could have gotten away with seeing her boyfriend by being more discreet. He said, "You are really making the decision when you force someone else to protect you, why not make the decision yourself? You are trying to make us do what *you* decided yourself. Since *you* are making the decision, really make it! I am going to leave you on privileges. If you need to be taken off privileges to help you handle the situation, just tell me and I'll take you off. The only advice I have for you is to be careful and not to get pregnant."

There are many possible sources of error. We can't know to what extent her verbal insights were accurate. The therapist made many assumptions. In at least one, he decided she meant the opposite of what she said. The statement that she wanted to stay on privileges was taken to mean she wanted to be taken off in order to demand that the therapist take care of her rather than push her into the world.

He assumed she was ready to make the decision overtly herself instead of in her customary way. The big assumption was that a great deal of self-confidence and personal integrity could be promoted by giving her responsibility *now* on something as obviously important as her affair. But the situation was problematical. What would be her husband's reactions if he found out about it? Should he be told what was being done? The boyfriend was unpredictable; he was a former patient himself who had been diagnosed as schizophrenic. How adequate were the clinical formulation and the constructs used to describe the patient? The outcome of the alternate decision of restricting ground privileges is impossible to know. From a scientific standpoint, an unbiased or unambiguous interpretation of the outcome is impossible.

Implicit in the decision of the therapist was the prediction that the patient would not have sexual relations with the boyfriend or even see him, would decide this herself, and would gain strength through the experience. The therapist gambled that the situation would be useful to the patient, providing it came out the way he anticipated. But from the standpoint of statistical prediction, the best bet was that those who can't follow the rules are not ready to have the responsibility to make the decisions which go with the freedom of ground privileges. Past experience had established, in a loose statistical sense, the rule of removing privileges to protect such patients.

One can look at the payoffs from the standpoint of the institution. What would have happened if the patient had become pregnant? One has to weigh the possible advantages and disadvantages not only to the patient, but to her husband, family, and also to the institution. What were the disadvantages of taking her off privileges? The therapist could have revoked the privileges and waited to do his experiment on a matter less crucial. Would therapy have been set back if she had been taken off privileges? How does one go about making such a decision? How does one place one's bets and evaluate the possible good with possible failure? What values could be used in this kind of decision? How much risk should an institution take? How much risk should a therapist expose a patient to? Are the values implicit in a health notion of mental illness? Finally, all of these questions falsely presuppose that one can make accurate estimates in order to justify the decisions. The concepts have not been verified. Given current practices, there is no simple way to evaluate the concepts, the formulation, or the logic of going from the formulation to the prediction.

This case, perhaps more than the others, illustrates the role of the formulation in making clinical decisions. It illustrates the importance of having an adequate conceptualization of a patient's behavior. It illustrates the need for having an adequate set of constructs to account for personality and for the particular symptoms the patient shows. It requires understanding which will allow us to predict accurately what will happen. Only when such understanding is sufficiently explicit to allow prediction can one have confidence in the formulation and make decisions about people. In short, we must be able to understand, predict, and control behavior before we have an adequate theory of psychopathology. But what concepts should we use for this task? The abstract and the practical meet head-on here.

The practicing clinician makes decisions like these many times a day—to restrict privileges or to give privileges; to discharge or to commit and so forth. Often decisions are made too quickly, but only because they must be made and someone has to do it. In the case just presented, the decision was made within an hour. Some action had to be taken by the therapist and any action implied a formulation and certain values.

One can ask if these decisions can be made intelligently when one man might be responsible for 300 or more patients. That is to complicate the problem with a different issue. The issue is indeed important. But the manpower is a separate question.

The current question is one of *verifiable knowledge*. How valid were the assumptions the therapist made in not revoking ground privileges? What right do we have to put confidence in our judgments, or alternatively speaking, how much confidence should we put in our judgments? How good are our theories?

9

clinical
decisions

Prediction is important at both the practical and the theoretical level. At the theoretical level, the verification of predictions lends greater under- standing of the nature of psychopathology. And on the practical side, accurate prediction is necessary to make useful decisions for the effective disposition of patients.

Clinical formulations have been illustrated by the examples given in the last chapter. In contrast is an actuarial approach which arrives at decisions about treatment of people on a statistical basis. The statistical approach can be illustrated by the task of predicting which prisoners can be successfully paroled and which cannot. To use a statistical approach, information is obtained about each one of a number of people who are eligible for parole. The information could be based on demographic data, such as socioeconomic class, or a score indicating relative standing on a personality dimension. It is determined empirically which items predict success or failure and the best way to weigh the information. The result is a prediction equation which yields a combined score which best predicts success and failure. A cut-off point is statistically arrived at which maximizes the number of correct decisions. For practical applications, the necessary individual scores are determined for each prisoner about whom decisions must be made, these are combined according to the equation and parole is granted or not depending on whether the final number is above or below the cut-off line. A table makes the decisions.

Empirical evidence

In order for the table to be useful, however, it must at least do better than *base rate expectancy*. In the case of parole violation, one study reports that the simple prediction of "successful" would be correct 56 per cent of the time. When a prediction equation was used combining personality measures and demographic data the accuracy could be raised to 63 per cent.[1]

Almost any kind of data can be used to construct a prediction equation, including clinical judgments. However, objective and empirically selected items are frequently used because they are easy to obtain and relatively reliable. Obviously, it would be of no value to use terms which prove unstable over time. For example, in the study just cited, the personality measures were taken from a test called the California Psychological Inventory. This test was developed by selecting groups of people who were similar in some respect, i.e., rated by peers as honest, steady, responsible, serious, industrious, modest, obliging, and sincere. Items were then found which separated these people from others, the result being a socialization scale. The entire test includes some eighteen separate scales, all empirically derived in the same way. Thus, the items which are used to differentiate between people with different characteristics are mechanically selected and thereafter used to arrive at a score on socialization, or one of the other seventeen characteristics, which is then used mechanically in a prediction equation.

The statistical approach offers an alternative to the clinical approach. Once tables are set up, the implementation can be left to clerks and automatic data-processing machines. Like the clinical, the statistical approach also requires classification of people into categories, both for empirical selection of items for the test and for application of the prediction equations. The nature of statistical or clinical prediction can be clarified by considering clinical prediction in a different light. If one examines the process whereby a clinician comes to make a decision, it appears that he must first decide what relevant facts he must know in order to have a basis for his decision. He must collect this information and then combine it in some fashion. Presumably, if the patient is impulsive and an unskilled laborer, he is figuring that the patient will break parole because such people frequently are out of work and have not been able to save money for periods of unemployment. The clinician must determine the attributes of the patient he deems to be crucial, and by so doing, he assigns the person to a class or locates him on a certain dimension. On the basis of his past experiences and inferences from theoretical notions (which serve the same purpose as a prediction equation) about how such individuals respond, he makes his prediction of the outcome and acts accordingly.

If 90 per cent of people who are impulsive and

unskilled break parole, then the clinician would also expect that of his particular case. If there is a rationale behind what the clinician does, if he is consistent with himself, if he uses rules that are based on his own experiences, and if the rules are probability statements on the likelihood of an outcome, then theoretically it is possible to make these rules systematic and be completely explicit about what information is to be obtained, how it is to be used, and the prediction it leads to. In short, the clinician is actually using statistical or actuarial predictions that he carries around in his head. There is much room for error, for there is no assurance that the clinician will remember accurately what needs to be remembered, or that he has sufficient basis for making his decisions, limited as he is by his own experiences and his own memory. Further, the clinician's own norms may not profit from empirical verification since, as we have seen, it is very difficult to know the outcome of many of the predictions and clinical decisions made on a day-to-day basis. Given the conclusion that the clinician is doing imperfectly what could be done statistically, it should be no surprise that statistical prediction even with simple elements exceeds the accuracy of clinical prediction.

Paul Meehl, a psychologist at the University of Minnesota, has reviewed the experimental literature contrasting the effectiveness of clinical versus statistical prediction.[2] Experienced clinicians were given clinical information which they combined by whatever logic and intuition they could muster to arrive at a prediction. Then the same data were combined statistically to arrive at a second set of predictions. In these experiments there was an objective outcome (criterion) known to the investigator which was obtained independently of the statistical or the clinical prediction. In the comparisons made, the statistical (frequently very simple statistical combinations of data such as giving equal weight to age, education, and a measure of adjustment) in every case, did just as well as (and in most cases, significantly better than), clinical prediction. It appears that the clinician could not give the proper weight to all of the factors or that he was led astray by some aspect of his formulation. This has been a negative contribution in the sense that it has shown the inadequacy of existing approaches but has not provided a usable alternative.

The fact that statistical prediction has come off relatively better than clinical does not, in fact, establish it as immediately more useful. Sufficient relevant tables do not exist in any satisfactory form and it is not clear that they can or will be developed. The parole study cited was a major undertaking. It resulted in a 7 per cent increase in accuracy above chance to 63 per cent, hardly an impressive showing, and only half of that increase was due to addition of personality variables to the simple demographic data.

Within the past two decades there have been an increasing number of professional workers who have questioned the usefulness of our traditional clinical assessment techniques and the adequacy of our concepts for understanding personality structure and dynamics. For the most part, these have been serious questions that cannot be ignored or overlooked. They are not attacks from critics who are unsympathetic to the practical and theoretical problems of personality assessment and psychopathology; but rather, they are reluctant expressions of disillusionment by many who have been concerned with clinical matters for many years. Their disillusionment is based on an ever-increasing body of research literature that suggests the *current clinical assessment-prediction techniques and their related concepts and principles of personality cannot be applied successfully for the*

125

WHAT'S WRONG WITH THE MENTAL HEALTH MOVEMENT

diagnosis, disposition and treatment of madness, or for the prediction of behavior in general.

Notable illustrations are the repeated failures of the Rorschach Test, one of the most widely used projective techniques, and of projective testing in general. In these tests, the patient either is shown a standard series of inkblots and is asked to describe what they remind him of, or an ambiguous picture and asked to tell a story about what is happening. It is assumed, because the stimulus has no clear characteristics, that the patient will project—read into the items—his own fears, motivations and personal style.

There is evidence that situational variance is a major contribution to the test data, and thus causes unwanted distortions. Transient and temporary stimuli which are present during testing may significantly influence the kind of assessment data obtained, and therefore influence the predictions or decisions arrived at clinically. For example, the sex of the examiner can significantly influence the kind of stories told on one of our most popular personality tests.[3] Mounting evidence shows that clinical judgment is little better than chance and usually poorer than statistical techniques. There is evidence that our assessment tests, when used in isolation, have generally poor prognostic value, and our projective techniques have been a failure methodologically and substantively in personality research.[4] More recent reviewers have been less harsh on some aspects of methodology but remain impressed by the practical failures.[5]

Essentially, the tone of these criticisms is that the clinical prediction and decision-making process is *completely unsatisfactory.* The evidence that clinical prediction can be beaten by very simple statistical procedures proves the relative failure. But there are absolute failures also. For example, the failure to exceed a base rate prediction; if it is known that 70 per cent of hospitalized psychotic

126

patients are schizophrenic, and if all patients were diagnosed as schizophrenic without looking at them, one could be just as accurate as if he had tried to pick out the seven who are and the three who are not schizophrenic. Put simply, a mistake is made 30 per cent of the time. With rarer events like suicide, one always fails to do as well as the base rates.

The need for the verifiable information recommended in the report of the Joint Commission is apparent. Progress can be made only when we can become more explicit and systematic about our theoretical notions and the ways in which they are to be applied. Yet, the day-by-day decisions that the practicing clinician makes cannot be bypassed. They cannot be avoided. They occur over and over again and, like it or not, someone has to decide on some basis.

Socio-Legal aspects

So far in this chapter we have contrasted the practical and theoretical, and in so doing have exposed a seeming incompatibility between the requirements for action and for science. In their own right, each perspective has its own priorities which can be given a relative ordering only by shifting to a different level of abstraction. This shift of levels is to the social value that man be judged by man and not by a flip of a coin, thus supporting the actions of mental health personnel. A deeper dilemma, however, then exists between this demand for action that must be taken and the political values implicit in our legal system which holds a person responsible for his behavior.

We have already considered some of the implications of involuntary hospitalization in the context of the social versus the medical nature of behavior disorders. The legal concept of insanity has some further implications, especially in relation to criminal acts.

Formerly, if a person did not know right from

wrong because he was mentally ill, he could be excused from *criminal* prosecution and would not be held *legally* responsible for his action. He would probably be held socially responsible and committed to a psychiatric hospital for treatment and would not be set free until he was deemed no longer mentally ill. In recent years, the American Psychiatric Association has pressed for and obtained a broader test which would hold the criminally accused not responsible, if the unlawful act were the product of mental disease or mental deficit. It is now possible for psychiatric testimony to take the form of a description of a defendant's mental state and personality. The psychiatrist may give an opinion about the presence or absence of mental illness and how it is related to the criminal act committed. The jury must then weigh this, along with other information, and decide if madness is present and criminal responsibility absent.

We have already considered the difficulty in specifying what are normal and therefore acceptable personality characteristics. We have just concluded a consideration of the difficulty in arriving at an adequate formulation or description of personality for prediction and decision; but in criminal cases, a formulation of the personality is required with respect to an absolute standard of normality and abnormality in order to decide whether a person, for instance someone who abused his child, should be held legally responsible for his criminal behavior. At present, these decisions must be made, since by law, insanity can be a condition excusing responsibility. If the person claims insanity then, in fact, it will be decided by the court if the person is or is not emotionally disturbed. To change current procedures would require a redefinition of madness and with it a major part of the role of the mental health expert.

The problem has many faces. There is the practical problem of making decisions, there is the scientific problem of the concepts to be used, and there is the humanistic problem of the values to be implemented. Unfortunately the faces cannot be considered separately, for the practical problem leads to actions which are incompatible with scientific and humanistic solutions. To the extent that an *action* creates problems concerning social values, it must be dealt with as such, rather than circumvented by mental health experts who wrap themselves in an infallible armor of absolute knowledge which ostensibly maintains their position as experts. The dilemma is felt by the social order also, for to confront madness from a humanistic or a scientific posture is to undermine the current basis for decisions that must be made each day.

The dilemma is not new or even unique to madness. It is important to confront the problem directly, however, because the resolution of the incompatibility by more sophisticated conceptual inventions is but another relative way to find truth. There will always be a point of friction, to be sure, but it is important to recognize where that point of contact is. In the case of madness the conceptual, the practical, and the moral aspects are distinguishable, but we have not yet found a way to face all three directly and simultaneously.

No single person can give completely satisfactory answers to the questions raised, for there are no definite answers. Although there may be no answers in any absolute sense, there are issues which are relevant to whatever answers are selected. Thus, by providing dimensions along which madness may be viewed, the range of possible conclusions will be limited.

Szasz has argued for publicly verifiable criteria for rendering judgments rather than the highly debatable opinions now given by expert witnesses. He has noted that contemporary psychiatry cannot provide a scientific distinction between mentally ill and mentally healthy persons. Szasz has concerned himself with the way the psychiatricization of the law may subvert the ethics of an open society by implicitly putting the goal of the good individual and public health above that of individual choice and responsibility. Szasz has concluded that the most dignified, and psychologically and socially most promising alternative is *not* to consider mental illness as an excusing condition in criminal court proceedings. He would treat offenders as responsible human beings even though sometimes they may not be individually blameworthy. This offers them the only chance, as he sees it, of remaining human and of possibly becoming more so. Szasz wishes, therefore, that the courts act as though *all people were responsible for their decisions.* Guided by a concern for an open society, Szasz's suggestion does not mean that the law would blindly ignore the circumstances of a crime, or that the courts would simply punish the criminal for his self-chosen wickedness, or that society would take no responsibility for madness as a social problem.

Szasz has questioned *the scientific defensibility* of the use of psychiatric formulations regarding important social aspects of human behavior. *We are here questioning the legitimacy of maintaining clinical formulations and decisions as proper answers to these important human problems.* As long as our formulations lack indication of their validity, it is misleading to allow them to determine in such an important way aspects of the social order and civil liberties.

Commentary

Through the practical demands of necessity, the adequacies and inadequacies of our theories and concepts are most vividly portrayed. Since formulation plays such a crucial role, it is necessary that we be open about the adequacy of our concepts and what they can and cannot do. Our concepts of madness historically reflect man's effort to deal with a social problem: religiously, medically, and now in mid-twentieth century, scientifically. The moral, health, and scientific approaches are not quite concerned with the same invention, but all reflect humanistic concern over a social problem.

Our dynamic theories of personality and psychopathology tend to be extremely flexible. This lack of logical cohesion means that we can never be as sure as we would like to be about the implications of a formulation, or even that the formulation itself is internally consistent. These kinds of problems are not unique to psychology or psychiatry. Their intensity perhaps reflects the arrival of a scientific approach to a new area of inquiry, particularly one that touches so directly on man's life and how he lives it. After all, acceptance of the idea that man could and should be permitted to study himself scientifically is not very old.

In the Middle Ages, man placed himself at the mercy of God; bounty and sickness, life and death were all beyond his control. But the Modern Age which followed has slowly replaced spiritual faith with the tenet that man can know the world through reason. The Age of Reason, like a wave, first slowly swelling and then rapidly breaking, has come rushing over us—through the transition from literature and logical analysis to science and technology, from bending the physical world to serve human needs, to treating man himself as just another object who is also subject to unyielding laws. Those of us alive today are standing at the threshold of perhaps the culmination of the Age of Reason, the last chapter of the Modern Age. Because the pace has now become so fast, we may, within our lifetime, see the end. It is for us to bear witness to the outcome of turning science and technology on ourselves. How well we fare will depend, in a large measure, on how we manage the role and place of the mental health movement.

The arrival of serious science, along with the rather unsuccessful record of dynamic approaches, has resulted in a fairly lively theoretical controversy about the kinds of concepts to be used. This controversy is, of course, abstract and far removed from the practical affairs of the world. The behavioral, in contrast to the dynamic approach, does not try to build a system of personality out of elements such as unconscious hostility or lovelessness. Rather, it tries to understand the ways in which certain acts are acquired. The extreme behavioral position looks at how man learns to be what he is, assuming that by using the processes of perception, learning, and motivation we can understand, predict and therefore have the possibility to control behavior. The dynamic and the behavioral are fundamentally different views.

What is to be proposed after all of this? The role of clinician cannot be given up and decisions cannot be postponed until there is an adequate science. Conceptual advancement can come only when competent people expose themselves to the realities of the dilemma with insight. The clinician is asked to approach his task with concern for his patient and for the practical demands to be met, but with an open and scientifically inquiring mind.

This openness is impeded by the role the mental health expert is establishing for himself—having the secret to mental health so as to give a periodic check-up like the dentist and to make social judgments about health or illness as if it were an absolute standard to be appealed to rather than a social concept. These are illustrations of selling a product that does not exist and creating a market for it by a commercial definition.

Clinicians collect fees from individuals in return for a product represented as science, which, if the clinician is honest with himself, does not allow him to be right very often. The need for self-justification, I believe, has led many clinicians to believe sincerely that they really do understand. Many of us who cannot convince ourselves that we know the answers engage in research which is often highly theoretical in nature and far removed from actual clinical conditions. This, in no small measure, contributes to the dichotomy that exists between the practicing (usually dynamic) aspects of psychology and abstract (often behavioral) research. The researcher is not faced with a ward of patients whose mere presence demands decisions.

The question at hand is not whether a clinical formulation is right or wrong. In the illustrations presented in the last chapter, the patient had either to be left on or taken off ground privileges; the depressed patient had to be discharged or committed; someone had to decide whether the lady who threw the hatchet could go home or not. Someone has to decide one way or the other and the decision is going to turn out either right or wrong. The important issue is to make decisions with full knowledge that the patient may become pregnant, that the patient may commit suicide, that the patient may bury the hatchet in her husband's head, or that someone else may be affected by the decision. We have no choice but to learn to live with these anxieties and, as professional workers or scientists, to take the responsibility with an open attitude of inquiry and effectively utilize the consequences for further advancement and understanding.

The viewpoint of madness presented here is not the one advertised by the National Association for Mental Health, which views mental illness and personality as akin to a carburetor on a car which, when it starts to malfunction somewhat, can be taken to a friendly psychiatrist for a tune-up. The problem is not that simple. Mental illness is not just a psychiatric and psychological problem; it includes many social, economic, moral, ethical, and legal complications that cannot be given simple answers, and most certainly cannot be solved by the limited perspective of the mental health expert alone. The general public should have a more realistic view of our so-called mental health problem; the realistic view is less comforting than what is advertised, but it is a view that will hopefully put the area of psychopathology into better perspective. The practical decisions must bear the burden of giving substance to theoretical abstractions. It is improper to hide problems of verification and to act as if the current solutions were a product of science, rather than to present behavioral disorders as social problems toward the solution of which science can make only a partial contribution.

10

psychotherapy

Most therapists are convinced that their efforts, at least with some of their patients, are highly successful. They believe that the psychotherapeutic process has effected many significant and long-lasting changes in individual patients. They publish case histories which illustrate the changes produced by some particular technique or procedure. For example, as Sigmund Freud did in describing how free association and later the analysis of dreams could be used to uncover repressed emotions and thereby cure hysterical symptoms. And more recently, how behavioral techniques, such as rewards of caramel candy for using the potty, can be used to modify behavior.[1] The achievement of effecting psychological well-being in others is self-evident to therapists on the basis of their personal experience.

However, the psychologist Paul Meehl has called the attention of therapists to the fact that *nonsystematic* observations and beliefs are not suitable as evidence.[2] There is no such thing as a self-evident outcome. We need to verify the accuracy of our observations and our beliefs using the available scientific criteria. The appeal to scientific verification is not a sacrifice of humanism to science. It means simply that we take precautions to be sure that what we believe to be self-evident is not actually otherwise. Scientific verification requires open-mindedness. Alternatives are to be considered or rejected according to rules.

We have no difficulty today in rejecting witchcraft for the simple reason that the concept of "witches" fails to meet acceptable standards as viable knowledge. Confessions obtained under duress are unacceptable evidence of guilt. Leading questions implying a desired answer are ruled out of order in our courts of law. Advice and reports by a person with a vested interest—be he an inquisitor or a used-car salesman—are regarded with suspicion lest he be misrepresenting his product for personal ends. Likewise, modern standards must be employed in the evaluation of psychotherapy. Illustrative case studies and personal observations alone are not sufficient.

One of the difficulties in evaluating the outcome of psychotherapy is obtaining an adequate indication of that outcome. For example, one could obtain a self-report from the patient as to whether he had been helped by the treatment. However, psychologists and psychiatrists are not always sure they want to trust this judgment on the part of the patient, just as they have been unwilling to accept it as the criterion for normality-abnormality. Can improvement be something an individual can know for himself? He may be bitter at having paid large sums of money to purchase his therapy, or he may be trying to reassure himself that his current improvement is at last permanent, and not merely another temporary repose as was the case on several previous times. Alternatively, one could obtain a rating by the therapist as to whether his patient was improved or not. But again this might be a biased report. The therapist, as well as the patient, has a personal investment in the outcome. The therapist has a product to sell, as does the used-car salesman. It is a product that is advertised through the offices of his professional association.

Further, it is not always clear what constitutes a treatment. Does one session count as a treatment or must it continue until one or both parties are satisfied? How long should a recovery last before it is counted as a cure? For example, if the number of patients discharged is counted, a cure would only have to last one day to be a success. Or should a cure last a year, or longer, before it is counted? If a patient stops therapy before the treatment is complete, as judged by the therapist, and has a relapse, is that a failure? But if the patient stays well, does that constitute success? At what point is a relapse a new sickness, and at what point is it a failure of the previous treatment? These are questions that have a bearing on the central question of whether or not psychotherapy effects changes in patients.

Much of the research that has been done in psychotherapy has assumed that the treatment itself was of value, and the object of the research was to show that some proportion of those treated showed permanent cures over some specified period of time. The effect of the treatment was assumed to be self-evident; the research question was not whether, but how effective the treatment was. Such assumptions cannot be made without checking whether or not they can be supported. There is a need to have a control group, which is a group of equivalent patients who are not given psychotherapy. Usually patients are randomly assigned to the treatment condition or to the control condition and are treated essentially the same in all respects except for receiving the treatment. If psychotherapy has any advantage, a greater proportion of persons who have been given psychotherapy should recover than those not receiving psychotherapy, and the recovery should be longer-lasting. In fact, troubled people have their ups and downs. If therapy goes on long enough, both parties are likely to attribute any improvement which occurs to the therapy, when in fact the two may be unrelated. The protection offered by hospitalization and the additional allowance made by others for the fact that the patient just "had a nervous breakdown" may be sufficient to account for whatever changes are taken as an index of cure.

The effects of psychotherapy

There have been two comprehensive reviews of the experimental literature on the effectiveness of psychotherapy, both done by the English psychologist H.J. Eysenck.[3] On this question, as on clinical formulations and decision-making, the usefulness of the concepts for understanding personality and psychopathology were on the line. We should be able to help people if the nature of madness and the personality process is understood. Our abstractions must have testable and practical implications. Eysenck reviewed a number of studies on the effectiveness of psychotherapy and he concluded that the burden of proof is on the practitioner who claims specific positive results for a given form of psychotherapy. When control groups are included, those patients recover to the same extent as those patients receiving treatment. The therapeutic effects of psychotherapy (excepting methods based on learning theory) did not add any improvement beyond that produced by the routine attention afforded all patients.

The enthusiastic belief expressed by therapists about their effectiveness, in spite of the negative results, illustrates the problem of the therapist who must make important human decisions many times each day. He is in a very awkward position unless he *believes* in what he is doing. On the other hand, it is misleading and, in the end, detrimental to the progress of science to insist on the correctness of that belief and thus to lose sight of the process of verification that must guide such endeavors.

Two aspects of Eysenck's review need to be considered. The first has to do with establishing the effectiveness of psychotherapy as a *criterion*. The second is the distinction between psychotherapy based on learning theory and techniques based on personality dynamics and the extent to which psychotherapy provides a *critical encounter* between these two alternatives (referred to here as the dynamic and behavioral).

Psychotherapy as a criterion

The outcome of success and failure in psychotherapy is by no means a straightforward affair. A gross criterion, such as the number of arrests accumulated by boys who as predelinquents were given extensive counseling, can be objected to as too general because it overlooks the personal impact the counselors may have had on the boys— that is, the effect of this human concern on the personal life of the boys. Yet a measure of the number of times the boys sought the advice of the counselor or expressed appreciation for help they received could be considered as trivial if it did not help them to stay out of trouble.

A criterion can be judged as suitable or not only by making assumptions at a different level. A therapist with a psychodynamic viewpoint may very well reject the number of arrests as unsuitable, but not the evidence that the contact was valued.

However, a behavioral therapist is likely to have the opposite view. What measures of the effectiveness of psychotherapy are suitable demands to place on those abstractions which claim to deal with mental illness?

Science, as we have seen, presents an incomplete perspective of madness because the practical aspects must offer the final proving ground for the abstractions. There must be an interplay between the abstract and the practical. To the extent that an abstraction has success on the practical proving grounds, it is rendered plausible, and in this sense the application leads the science as well as follows it.

The need for an adequate criterion represents the convergence of the demands provided by the limited perspectives of both the abstract and the practical. The lack of effectiveness of dynamic psychotherapy renders it unsalable as a product of science, but not necessarily sterile as an idea. Concepts behind a technological failure must be returned to the science for reevaluation. An individual scientist may hold to them still, and his fame and fortune will ride on the wisdom of his choice. The technology, however, is bound to the ethics of the Better Business Bureau and should not be sold without verification. The mental health expert, however, is selling a product that can be justified only in the limited perspective of science.

Relying on my own feelings and my own observations, I am fully convinced that I have caused important, lasting and constructive changes in individual cases. But I have no independent verification that these people would not have changed in the same way if left to their own devices. The use of selected cases as validation continues to be the clinical tradition. The conclusions I reached out of my own personal experience cannot be accepted as valid evidence for the effectiveness of my treatment procedures or for the adequacy of my theories. So it was with the Grand Inquisition; so it is now.

Psychotherapy as a critical encounter

In his review of the literature on the effectiveness of psychotherapy, Eysenck noted that the only exception to the negative results may be treatment based on learning theory. This competitive alternative cannot be ignored, even though it strips the clinician of his role as mental health expert. Rather, it places him in the role of having knowledge—based primarily on principles of learning theory—which *may be* used toward socially defined ends. No claims inherent in the knowledge justify defining what is appropriate behavior.

The behavior alternative seeks to *use* psychology to effect changes in behavior. It provides no language for categorizing people into types and categories or for enumerating a list of personality traits; it describes *how* people learn to do and feel as they do, and thereby it provides a technology for changing behavior. The behavioral approach makes no pretense to be a theory of madness—it is a theory of behavior regardless of the content of the behavior.

If we contrast the two approaches, we see on one hand the traditional dynamic-personality view attempting to find a formulation of the personality and to rebuild the personality to do away with the source of the anxiety. On the other hand, the behavioral alternative will simply note that the patient is fearful; the treatment technique is straightforward and simple, because anxiety is a response which can be modified. The deconditioning procedure, developed by Joseph Wolpe, takes perhaps a dozen sessions, and the patient is freed of the anxiety.[4] No assumption is made about the underlying personality, nor is there a need to invoke concepts such as repressed hostility, fixation at some level of psychosexual development, or sexual feelings toward a parent of the opposite sex, to mention a few of the more popular concepts. The behavioral techniques simply utilize known empirical procedures to effect changes in behavior. Such a viewpoint makes the problem of clinical formulation partially obsolete since it reduces some of the necessity for the kinds of clinical concepts we now use. But this behavioral approach has its own limitations; it does not apply to a large number of the daily problems with which a practicing clinician must deal.

The view of man is different. The role of the mental health expert is different. The relationship of the practical to the abstract is different. The definition of madness is different. The field of psychology and its organization into various sub-specialties are different. The criterion of evaluation and the standards for training are different. The dynamic and behavioral alternatives are representative of many fundamental issues and problems of psychology. To an important degree the relative effectiveness of psychotherapy is an important critical encounter for these issues and problems.

An illustrative case history

The problem can be illustrated by a case history. One patient was hospitalized with a phobia about handling anything sharp. She could not use a pair of scissors, a knitting needle, a knife, or even a potato peeler. Her fears kept her out of the kitchen, incapacitating her as a wife and mother. She felt extremely unhappy about the difficulty that her foolish behavior was causing her family. She received a form of desensitization treatment known as reciprocal inhibition. Following Wolpe's methods, a list was made of the items which frightened the patient. At the top of the list were items which brought about acute distress and at the bottom of the list were things which aroused little fear, for example, a picture of a plastic toy knife. The patient was given relaxation exercises because relaxation is a state incompatible with anxiety. While relaxed, she was systematically exposed to the list of items, starting at the bottom. After she could stay relaxed while looking at a picture of the plastic toy knife, the next item was introduced, and so on progressively through the list. Soon she was able to remain relaxed while handling toy knives and scissors. Within a dozen sessions, she had been desensitized and was able to handle the real items while remaining relaxed. The anxiety was gone, and the patient was discharged back to her home. At a six-month follow-up she was doing well and by her own report was satisfied and happy. The report was confirmed by her husband and children. Here is an illustration of a cure, achieved in twelve sessions. It was a cure in the sense that the patient's symptoms were no longer present and showed no signs of returning.

Consider the case from the alternative psychodynamic point of view. The dynamic orientation would probably reject the treatment as a *cure* because there was something wrong within the personality that was not corrected. It is assumed that if there is something wrong with the personality, it cannot be remedied merely by treating a symptom, for the underlying defect remains. To cure a disorder, one must treat the personality. This is an assumption, of course, and the justification depends upon such things as the relative effectiveness of the treatment.

The patient was also given a traditional clinical formulation from a psychodynamic point of view. Her life history was taken in detail and a clinical formulation was constructed. It was discovered that she was an educated, hard-working, ambitious woman. Throughout her life she had known success and achieved whatever she attempted. Her parents had been very strict, and she had a strong moral upbringing. As an adult, much of her behavior followed principles dictated by the values of her conscience. She was responsible, reliable, meticulous, fair, and just. She married a man who was probably not as bright as she and who seemed to lack her self-disciplined drive and ambition. Note that none of this information can be regarded as fact. It is an *inference* made after collecting the case-history data. The information might be biased by what the clinician thought he should find, by the nature of the questions he asked, or by what the patient thought she should say. Or assuming these distortions were absent, we have no way of assessing their accuracy, for the information is clearly a retrospective report of her life and her personality development from the unusual vantage point of being a patient.

The psychodynamic reconstruction which follows will allow the reader to see the nature of clinical formulation and the inferences and assumptions which were made.

Apparently, the patient's husband never lived up to her ideal; he never achieved what she felt she could have achieved if she had had his opportunity and freedom. She felt that the responsibilities of being wife and mother forced her to stay at home. It would have been morally wrong from her value system to work or pursue a career of her own—it would be equivalent to deserting her children. However, underneath these demands of conscience were unconscious feelings of resentment and hostility toward her husband. He had imprisoned her. If it had not been for him, she could be out in the world achieving more than he and making a better living. She felt unconscious hostility toward him for not being a better provider; she was without the comforts she would have liked to have had and most of her friends enjoyed. There was resentment and dissatisfaction with her role as wife and mother, but an inability *to admit to herself* she was unhappy or dissatisfied, or to express her hostility directly toward her husband. The term "unconscious" is used because the patient explicitly denied the validity of the interpretation given. As her unconscious hostility came closer to becoming obvious to her—as the impulses, the resentment, the anger, and the frustration came closer to breaking out into the open—psychological defenses came into play. The woman had to protect herself from these hostile and aggressive impulses toward her husband in order to retain the image of herself as a worthy wife and mother. Any sharp instrument, such as a knife or a pair of scissors, could effect destruction and could be used, for example, to kill her husband. Such a thought would evoke tremendous anxiety in this person; she had to defend herself psychologically.

Her kind of personality structure is ideal for development of a phobic defense. In this case, staying away from objects which could be used to harm her husband or children because they imprisoned her in an inescapable situation, allowed the woman to control effectively the anxiety caused by her own hostile impulses. The fear and anxiety aroused by the objects of the phobia provided a diversion by requiring the patient to arrange her life so as never to come into contact with those items. In the early stages, the problem of shopping for food that could be prepared without the use of a sharp utensil was an exacting and absorbing demand which soon proved impossible. The mere mechanics of arranging the world so that a phobic patient can get by consumes an impossible amount of energy. The amount of energy so consumed is another aspect of the defense.

Such was the dynamic formulation of the patient's problem. The invention was carefully arrived at using dynamic personality theory, projective tests, and case history data. To treat the patient dynamically would require a reconstruction of her personality. Treatment would require that the patient probe her past experiences to gain insight. She would have to be able to recognize the conflict between her values and her emotions. She would have to recognize both of her conflicting wishes: to be a good mother and to avoid being imprisoned in her home. She would have to recognize her responsibilities and positive feelings toward her husband, and her simultaneous hostility and resentment toward him for failing to meet her standards. Once the ambivalent feelings and emotions were out in the open, the patient would then be in a position to consider their sources in order to strip them of the irrational emotional components of childhood origin. Then she would be in a position to reconsider her values—that a mother needs to be at home—and her responsibilities, and perhaps emerge from this experience with a different kind of personality structure; one freed from the uncompromising demands of a strong conscience, but aware of her own and her husband's needs.

Consider, however, the implications of this kind of major reconstruction, the hundred or so hours which are involved in a face-to-face encounter between the patient and the therapist. It would take time to lead this woman sympathetically so that she would verbally and consciously discover the conflict described. It takes time to get her conflict into the open, and then deal with it in a rational way. Would the woman have the patience to follow through with the task? I can imagine, for example, that once the conflict was in the open, the patient might get involved in an extensive examination of her personal values and her philosophy of life. A great deal of time might be spent on what should be the proper role of a wife and mother and on what is morally right and wrong. In traditional terms, the whole superego would have to be reconstructed and a new value system worked out, which would take a great deal of time and energy and be a painful process. We do not cast aside something as important as our values and replace them with an alternative at the drop of a hat or with only conversation in an office. To change any significant part of ourselves is to change our whole self. The implementations must be translated into new behavior never tried before. When one part of the personality structure is changed, it has reverberations throughout the whole business of day-to-day living.

Her values concerning the pursuit of her own career as a working mother would end up with reverberations in moral issues of good and bad, and would require considerable effort to work through. The patient might experience many anxieties and discomforts, be unhappy, cry, and worry while much of this was happening. The recovery might be hard on her children and her husband in terms of the financial drain required for the prolonged period of therapy. The cost might make the husband feel more inadequate for his failure to provide and in turn make the wife even more angry at the husband and make her feel that he is even more inadequate.

The patient would have to deal with her dissatisfaction in her selection of a husband. She would have to deal with the feeling that she could have achieved more than he, given the freedom he had. Maybe she would decide, after working these feelings through, that she had made a mistake and should not have married him. Maybe the new personality cannot live with the husband that the old personality selected, or the husband with his wife's new personality. One implication of prolonged psychotherapy might be the decision that she had made a mistake and that she should divorce this husband. But, does she owe her husband and family something, especially after they suffered hardships to provide the $2,000 to $3,000 needed for therapy and

147

stood behind her while she was distressed by her insights? Now we are engaged in another battle of values and conscience.

It is clear to me how traditional psychotherapy based on our dynamic theories of personality and psychopathology could be ineffective and in the long run harmful. I can conceive how behavorial approaches, which ignore the personality formulation and treat only the symptoms at hand, could with respect to all objective criteria yield better and more permanent results. It is easy to see how the twelve-session cure of the phobia may be a superior form of treatment; it is not difficult to see how our traditional forms of psychotherapy may be no more effective than being given patient status by receiving only routine medical attention or no treatment at all. Indeed, the traditional forms may be disruptive and cause as many new problems as they are able to produce cures.

This comparison is all very hypothetical, of course. The same case cannot be treated twice in order to experiment. Several implicit points can be noted. The dynamic approach necessarily becomes involved in the problem of the patient's morals and values. The case at hand could not be treated without touching on the patient's personal philosophy of life. How can a mental health expert deal in these commodities as an example of *scientific knowledge,* of a mental *illness,* or as a state of the organism to be assessed by a periodic check-up as some psychiatrists have suggested? These are not medical problems as much as they are social problems—at least at the applied level. At the level of perspective provided by science a wider range of ideas can be entertained, but they are not now marketable commodities.

The case also illustrates the problem of defining what is meant by a cure. What outcome could be classified as an effective cure? What should be required in order to say that this woman has been cured? Whose value system or implicit view of man is to be used to arrive at this decision? The effectiveness of psychotherapy can be evaluated only by making some initial judgments about a criterion, which implies a decision about the very issues to be investigated. Science is an arbitrary process in many respects.

The relationship between a theory and what is considered an acceptable criterion is illustrated by the notion of cure. From a dynamic framework, hostility toward the husband was a causal factor and a cure necessarily must deal with this fundamental characteristic. The dynamic framework would question what happened to the hostility after the behavioral cure. But, unconscious hostility is a problem only for the dynamic viewpoint, not for the behavioral viewpoint. Once reconceptualized from the behavioral viewpoint, *unconscious hostility no longer exists.* Concepts are inventions, and unconscious hostility is a concept, not something inside the patient. It should be put there only if it is more useful to do so than not to do so.

A shift in levels of explanation often makes it impossible to compare meaningfully the two alternative ways for viewing a person. One can only ask which is more useful for permitting prediction and control. The dynamic view would anticipate symptom substitution, which did not in this case occur. The behavioral view eliminated a complaint and produced a person who again could peel potatoes and say she was happy. The dynamic wants to repair an internal balance so that an unconscious force does not erupt, the behavioral wants to use information to produce desired behavior. The former treats mental illness, the latter tries to control behavior using whatever information is available, including medical (biological) and psychological concepts.

The technology of treating madness must pass

the fallible but existing criterion of verification. Science provides the rules for this verification and the basis on which a technology may be built. The report of the Joint Commission calling for more verifiable knowledge rests on the belief that a solution to the problem of madness falls heavily on increased knowledge about man. The way we will use the information of the behavioral sciences raises important *practical* and *ethical* and *scientific* questions. The practical aspect concerns what can be done for or to others; the ethical aspect concerns the grounds for doing so; and the scientific aspect concerns the nature of the abstractions that can be used to arrive at a more comprehensive scheme for understanding, predicting, and controlling the behavior of man.

11

an
overview

To a large extent, what follows is the raison d'être of this book. An overview will be given in this chapter, to be followed by a consideration of community mental health, the most recent expansion of the mental health movement into society, and finally by prescriptions for future action. The last three chapters look toward the future and the options still available.

The humanistic marketplace

It is now clear that there exists a large and growing psychiatric - psychological marketplace. There is a consumer demand for the product called happiness. Happiness has become a right and the lack of it cause for introspection and self-doubt. Larger, in terms of human suffering, but less visible, are the 1.2 million people each year who find their way into, and often out of, psychiatric hospitals. The psychiatric hospitals are the ignored aspects of abnormal psychology. They have existed in more or less the same form for the last fifty years and represent the old, not the new and growing, marketplace.

The expanding marketplace has grown well beyond severe psychopathology. The enlightened parent now raises his child in the psychologically correct way. Bettelheim with his psychodynamic concepts of personality is a rival to the more traditional views of Dr. Spock as a guide to good motherhood. The tremendous market for popularized psychology is illustrated by the immediate success of the magazine *Psychology Today.* The most popular magazines ranging from the intellectual to the woman's variety all contain psychiatric articles with explicit advice on how to live with yourself, your children, and your mate. There are checklists for this or that aspect of living. The oedipal situation is accepted as fact by many semi-popular writers as are numerous other concepts from dynamic (usually psychoanalytic) psychiatry, which increasingly forms the basis for novels, plays, and literary reviews. Knowing about psychiatry is the way to be sophisticated and enlightened.

But the marketplace is even larger than mental illness, adjustment, and semipopular and popular literature. Society seems convinced that its social troubles are really mental health problems, such as the violence, civil disobedience, and riots of the 1960s. The *understanding,* the *causes,* and the implication for *actions* have been conceptualized in such psychological terms as frustration, the failure to identify, the absence of socializing conditions necessary for the internalization of conscience and social responsibility, and so on. Modern America has accepted psychiatric and psychological levels of explanation as suitable and appropriate ways to approach its many social problems. The acceptance is illustrated by the formal reliance courts now place on psychiatric and psychological testimony; as in the decision of the Iowa Supreme Court to refuse a natural father custody of his son in favor of elderly maternal grandparents who took care of the boy after the mother was killed in an automobile accident. The father maintained contact with his son while relocating on the west coast. After establishing a new home he wished to take care of his son, but the grandfather objected. The reason given by the court for its decision, based on psychiatric testimony, was that the boy had formed a positive masculine identification with the grandfather and that his personality development would be damaged by separation.[1]

There are reasons for the existence of this marketplace. To a certain extent, the mental health product has been oversold to modern America by the American Psychiatric Association and by the American Psychological Association, to mention only two organizations. These and other professional groups have successfully hawked a product to a receptive public, and have acted in the spirit of guilds and trade unions to restrict practice to those certified by the guild in order to insure the public that practitioners have been carefully trained. The product has been sold to the public as a discovery of medical science to be benevolently dispensed by experts who understand psychological health and who promise to alleviate individual and social problems by their understanding.

The behavioral sciences—including psychology—undoubtedly will have important contributions to make in the next decade or two about many problems of humanistic concern. It is probably useful to look at urban riots and social problems from the level of explanation that can be provided by psychology, just as it is fruitful to look at them from other levels of explanation—such as economic and sociological ones—to see what implications follow from other views. The problems are multi-dimensional, and different levels of explanation will undoubtedly have different areas of convenience and usefulness. The use of this information, however, is a social matter and a problem for society as a whole. Science will tell ways to accomplish certain ends but not what these ends should be. The particular purposes such information may be put to, however, touch man in a way that goes beyond the contribution of the discipline which provided the information.

The use of psychology is neither good nor bad, neither right nor wrong. It has become a fact of life. As information (useful levels of explanation) about man becomes available it will be put to work for better or for worse. But, the purposes to which information will be put are not dictated by the science.

In the context of the here and now, we have mental health experts who claim that there is now a view of man that rests not on fleeting social values but on scientific knowledge. The mental health expert will now sell this new-found discovery of the nature of man which permits the problem of madness to be seen as an illness, an illness that can be cured. Verifiable knowledge is the product being sold by the mental health movement. From it follows the possibility of an absolute definition, a health or sick distinction, a psychiatric fit or unfit evaluation, and the once-a-year psychiatric check-up.

There are, however, conflicting claims. The psychodynamic views sells what it claims is a product of science. The counterclaim is that the dynamic view is not a technology derived from science because it has not met minimum standards of verifiable knowledge. Therefore, it is said, the mental health expert is a fraudulent businessman capitalizing on widely felt social problems. This counterclaim does not deny the need for concern over the problems the mental health expert deals with, but attempts to reexamine the basis for concern and to open inquiry as to whether existing procedures are appropriate to the social needs. The dynamic view of man has recently come under fire by an alternative, the behavioral view, which claims scientific respectability for the technology it is producing.

Foundations for a dynamic technology

If the mental health movement in its current form is to be acceptable and to be true to its own claim, it must provide evidence for the verifiability of its prescriptions. In view of the material presented—on diagnosis, psychotherapy, the definition of normality, legal testimony, and psychiatric formulations and decisions—one must question where this evidence is to originate and what form it is to take.

Established psychiatrists have also critically examined where the proof for psychodynamic concepts is to be found. Their conclusion, and ours, is simply that it is lacking. They note the failure of psychotherapy, as we did in our consideration of it as a critical encounter. They note that therapy based upon psychoanalytic theory appears to produce change at about the same rate (or slower) as other persuaders, such as faith healing.[2]

The failure of the psychoanalytic approach in particular and psychodynamic approaches in general, has occurred at every turn. Society has been sold a scientific approach to behavior which is unacceptable as science. Unverified concepts about man should not be sold and actively promoted. Faith in a benevolent professional group is not enough, especially when the method of training and entrance into the professional guild of mental health experts is considered.

The training methods of the psychodynamic approach involve an apprenticeship under an established and recognized authority. Frequently this requires undergoing psychotherapy or psychoanalysis oneself—called a training analysis—to see further proofs of the concepts. The illustrative case history in this instance is one's self. Completion of the task is the requirement for final peer approval. Obviously there is a certain amount of pressure to discover the truth—to use a term from a different era—including the right to pursue one's career. It must be remembered that the professions control access to their field through admissions to the professional schools, through training, and ultimately through certification and peer regulation.

The mental health guild has more in common with trade unions and private clubs than it does with either science or man and his problems. In 1971, the Illinois Psychological Association, composed largely of professional psychologists, was disturbed by the fact that the Illinois Psychiatric Association and Medical Society were using their lobby to attempt to defeat in the Illinois legislature the psychologists' freedom-of-choice legislation. The psychiatrists were accused of pursuing a "protectionist policy designed for their own economic advantage." The freedom of choice legislation would mandate that, in addition to psychiatrists, registered psychologists (but not other mental health workers) would receive reimbursement when consulted by patients covered under group-health-insurance plans. Psychiatrists wished to retain this right solely for themselves. The Illinois Psychological Association was appealing for donations to help the lobby effort; both groups had already spent considerable money. The title "freedom of choice" is itself somewhat of a misnomer, but the picture of two professional associations fighting for insurance spoils should leave no doubt as to the guild aspect of the professions and their basically antiprogressive and proeconomic function.

Little in the training procedures or in the organized actions of the American Medical Association, the American Psychiatric Association, or the professional branch of the American Psychological Association indicates that they are scientific groups. Rather, they are professional groups vigorously defending vested interests of an economic nature. Contrary to the values of an open and free society, such professional groups will make decisions regarding social values as if the information were verified. The training procedure insures that the "truths" which are popularly propagated are perpetuated, and the questioning necessary for an open-minded inquiry and advancement of knowledge is effectively made difficult. The ingredients most necessary to justify the label "science" are absent. The ingredients which are present bespeak of trade union, guild, or private club.

Foundations for behavioral science

The behavioral method, and the view of man it implies, is a different set of concepts for approaching the study of behavior. The approach started in the laboratory and has been most concerned with being accurate and precise. The guiding belief is that only through adequately developed concepts can one build knowledge. The view has grown into an approach that does not employ descriptive personality characteristics, but rather attempts to specify the process and conditions under which various behaviors will occur. The goal is simply to invent ideas and concepts relevant to human behavior which will allow us to make "if this, then that" types of statements.

WHAT'S WRONG WITH THE MENTAL HEALTH MOVEMENT

Proof has been largely an internal matter for the behavioral science approach. It has retained the limited perspective of science. The steps are to take any reliable phenomenon, to invent ideas to account for it, to derive further implications from these ideas, to test them empirically in situations where the ideas may be disproved, to elaborate the ideas, to do more tests for *predictive* verification, in a never-ending circle.

The behavioral-science approach, as contrasted with the dynamic, is an alternate way to view man. This different posture taken toward the nature of behavior has begun to yield a different technological approach to madness. To be justified on the market, it must meet a criterion of usefulness. And the usefulness itself also will bear further evidence on the adequacy of the concepts of the behavioral science approach to man. The proof is not yet in. The available data show a relative superiority of the behavioral science technology versus the dynamic technology.

Just as with the dynamic approach, the behavioral approach also has its private club and, to some extent, guild. The requirements, however, are different from those required by the dynamic guild. Membership into the select circles of this science club requires one to demonstrate the capacity to use the rules of science. Frequently the demonstration is in terms of precisely controlled experiments. Built into the training procedure is respect for impartiality and objectivity. A questioning and critical attitude is highly valued. It is necessary not only to evaluate concepts, but it is considered a legitimate activity to question the rules for questioning the concepts. Terms such as academic freedom have their importance in contributing to an atmosphere that actively encourages open and free inquiry. New and controversial ideas are welcome. These qualities are sorely lacking in the dynamic approach, but they are the very qualities that must be upheld if a scientific orientation is to provide the basis for an emerging and progressively more useful technology.

The aesthetic picture of the behavioral alternative as the search for relative knowledge and truth with a standard of excellence as the sole standard is overidealized. The club has its guild aspects too; these have been kept small in the past because concern with practical matters has tarnished its image. However, now that there are strong efforts toward a technology, and new demands for relevance, the pressures of the commercial marketplace are placing new stress on the virtues which the behavioral has enjoyed over the dynamic. There is now the emergence of a *radical behaviorism* with overstated claims by a zealous reformation group which poses the distinct possibility of a new professional guild seeking to establish a self-defined position for the benefit and protection of man. The image of a Benevolent Association of Behavioral Engineers is no more satisfactory that the current propaganda to accept the American Psychiatric Association as the benevolent keepers of the nation's mental health. The problems posed by behavioral engineers are different than the ones posed by mental health experts, but they are also ones that need to be attended to in this period of transition.

Alternative moral and ethical problems

A further implication of the alternate views of madness and the technologies which they embody is the unique moral and ethical issues each presents. The behavioral alternative proposes to do things to people. It is a case of applying information from the behavioral sciences to effect certain desired changes in the behavior of others. There is no suggestion that their behavior is any different in principle than the behavior of nonpatients. Indeed, social values determine whose behavior is defined as acceptable (normal) or unacceptable (abnormal). Under these conditions, the behavioral engineer is working for someone to effect changes desired by society, by the patient, or by someone else. He uses psychology to effect changes in behavior that are defined as desirable on grounds other than the psychological principles used for controlling behavior. This technology creates the moral and ethical problem of the guidelines under which such information and procedures can be applied and used.

The psychodynamic alternative, however, creates a different set of moral and ethical problems. This approach is based on a health-illness view of madness from which some absolute statement can be given about the relative adjustment of an individual. Implicit in the definition of mental illness is a judgment made by a mental health expert. As we have seen, under these conditions the mental health expert may make decisions that directly or indirectly involve deprivation of freedom (involuntary hospitalization), civil liberties, criminal responsibility, and most frequently a changing of the nature of the person's philosophy of life (values). This approach touches on the personal values of individuals as well as on social, economic, and political values reflected in the concept of an adjusted or maladjusted personality.

The behavioral alternative

The technology that can be derived from a behavioral science foundation, i.e., the information and theories developed in the laboratory, is used to effect changes in matters of social concern. In this sense, there is a technology. The adequacy with which these concepts can be applied to the solution of humanistic problems will ultimately have bearing on the nature of the concepts and ideas we have for viewing man. However, with the development of a behavioral technology there arises a unique set of moral and ethical problems. These problems have not been faced directly before, because society has not been confronted with the dilemma behavioral technology poses. The questions that must be answered are by what authority, and by whom, is the information used to effect changes deemed desirable?

Efforts to change and influence behavior are, of course, hardly a new problem. Consider, for example, the proselytizing efforts of major religious groups. Think of the strenuous efforts of advertising people to induce consumers to desire certain products. What about the efforts of an army to get information or confessions of war crimes from its captives? These are all efforts to modify or influence behavior. Although wide varieties of techniques have been used, some are considered morally wrong. We have invented codes of "good" business practice, and advertisers are now prohibited from blatantly misrepresenting products, and it is "illegal" to torture war captives. These are efforts to restrict the variety of techniques and procedures used to modify or influence behavior.

Now another kind of behavior modifier comes along. He is called a behavioral engineer. With respect to madness, he openly and publicly admits that there is no way to define it and no reason to be especially concerned with the definition. He does say that madness is not an illness in the sense that it is a deviation from biological norms or a psychological state that can be identified and categorized by an expert. Instead the behavior modifier looks at madness as a manifestation of behavior and, as such, he treats it like any other behavior.

Presumably madness is a behavior that follows the same laws and is susceptible to the same principles that govern all of human behavior. From an ethical and moral point of view, the problem becomes a definition of what behavior is to be called mad and under what conditions. What steps will society take to do something to, or for, those people with or without their consent? The moral and ethical guidelines have not yet been set down. But if society is to deal with the moral dilemma presented by the behavioral sciences, the time to do it is now.

The threat the behavioral alternative poses is that of a new expert who would use his version of what is good to save the world. The visions of behavioral technologists are to program child-rearing to exclude unhappiness, to raise people who can love only, and to train people to enjoy certain skills in the exact proportion these skills are needed by society at large. It is a "brave new world" indeed. Sooner or later, society will have to face the problem of behavior control. But the particular decisions which need to be made are social, political, and economic. They are *not* primarily psychological in nature.

Indeed, the behavioral technologist may well expect to play an influential role in how these decisions are made. But beware, for the decisions are of a social nature. They are ethical and moral problems of society. They are not implicit in a science or technology of man. But technology may provide the *means* by which man will be confronted with new and important moral, ethical, and social questions. Yet, if these problems of values are given an absolute answer by behavioral technologists, then they will be assuming moral and ethical responsibilities. The behavioral engineering of radical behaviorism is an emerging threat to a free and open society, taking over the role currently occupied by the mental health expert.

The dynamic alternative

The dynamic alternative has its own set of moral and ethical problems. Perhaps the most serious of these is its false claims for effectiveness when such proof is lacking. The dynamic alternative is selling a product which does not exist. There can be no objection to the dynamic view of man as an abstraction, i.e., as a conceptual invention for academic thought, but it can be objected to on ethical grounds for selling mental health to the public as a verified product of science.

The second moral and ethical problem is related to the first. This is the presence of absolutes. An illness view carries with it the implication that there is a correct and an incorrect, or a good and a bad way, for a person to be (not necessarily behave). This view implies that there is an absolute standard of adjustment against which madness and behavior in general can be assessed. As such, it provides a philosophy of life and a prescription for living. What values, what behavior, what feelings, what emotions, what actions, what interpersonal relationships, what self-concepts, should a man with good mental health have? The dynamic approach, and its correlated illness view of madness, carries with it an implicit absolute standard of behavior. To accept the current definition of madness is to put into the hands of the mental health experts responsibility for decisions about moral and ethical matters of significant social consequence.

Commentary

If one accepts an "illness" viewpoint and a dynamic approach to madness, then one is accepting a view of man which has implicit standards for conduct. With the behavioral approach such standards would not exist. If the dynamic theorist's position is granted, then he can proceed with relatively few moral problems or little difficulty in implementing something for the good of society. If one makes an option for the behavioral camp, then the dynamic mental-health expert appears as a

163

fraudulent misrepresentative of science who has established a position for himself, and who, in the process, has gained access to power to make important decisions about how life should be lived. In a behavioral context, madness is no more a health problem than war, poverty, race relations, or lack of opportunity. Rather, these are social problems toward which various disciplines may have useful information for a solution. Psychology, through ways to modify behavior of individuals, presents itself to the social problem of madness.

The use of psychological and biological information about the nature of man toward the ends of social well-being—whatever that is—are worthwhile goals by themselves. Misrepresentation of knowledge where none exists, however, is detrimental to the accumulation of new information and to society's making sensible judgments about the problem. The easy solution of abandoning the problem to the judgment of mental-health experts or possibly to the behavioral engineers of *radical behaviorism* is an escape from freedom and a failure to use science for positive purposes.

A biological level of explanation will surely be one of the more important components of our more complete theory of man. But there is nothing within a biological level of explanation, any more than within a psychological level, that gives one power to make decisions about how people should live. When our theories become more precise, there may indeed be information which makes it easier to value one kind of behavior over another, but that information does not now exist. The word "illness" is too restrictive, for it puts weight on biological or psychological norms that do not exist.

The moral questions that we face are what society should do to whom, and under what conditions. The technological question is how to achieve this. It is improper and wrong to presume that a particular technology has implicit within it, standards for the appropriateness of behavior. At a scientific level, the behavioral and the dynamic alternatives represent two competing approaches to view man.

12

community
psychology

The mental health movement has now taken a new direction that considerably enlarges its scope. The concept of community mental health has provided the rationalization for this expansion, and community mental health projects and training programs are its actualization. A variety of factors have contributed to the emergence of this new mental health movement.

The Joint Commission Report of 1961 provided a compelling documentation of the need for widespread improvement in the mental health field. In 1963, President Kennedy gave high priority to mental health services and called for treatment within the patient's own community. Late in 1963, in response to the president's speech, the Community

Mental Health Centers Act was passed, providing $150 million for the construction of such centers between 1965 and 1967, as well as $224 million to staff these new facilities. In 1967, under President Johnson, the act was extended for the years 1968-1970, and an additional $238 million was allotted for centers and staff.

Although these special programs expired under President Nixon, the centers themselves continue as partial replacements for the services provided by the older and larger state hospitals. The goal is to treat the patient more intensively, but on a short term basis, close to his work, home, family, and friends where follow-up is possible. It was felt the smaller local center could respond better to the unique problems and nature of the community, gain local support, and serve as a prevention as well as a treatment function.

The establishment of these community mental health centers and the demands for staff provided the physical and financial impetus for professional expansion of social psychiatry and community psychology. Also important were ideological events which provided the supporting conceptual framework. The Joint Commission Report, and the legislation which followed, acknowledged a widespread need for mental health services. The urban riots, the youth rebellion, and the social problems which surfaced in public awareness during the late 1960s contributed to a felt need for some kind of solution. Many were proposed.

One was the need for law and order and another was called the *mental health solution.*

The new solution was to bring mental health to the community itself. Since there were too few professionals to deal with the problem, the solution was to take preventive steps. Preventive therapy would thereby reduce the number of people who became disturbed by curing the social problems that

168

contributed to mental illness. The analogy was made that typhoid fever was never brought under control by treating individual cases, but rather by removing the cause. Thus, community mental health was seen as being similar to preventive medicine. Psychology and psychiatry should, according to the new ideology, actively move into the community. Its early intervention would promote positive mental health by dealing with the predisposing conditions.

Community psychology has been able to give a broader definition to the community mental health ideology than has social psychiatry, in part because psychology is relatively free from the mental illness concept and medical analogy. But also because the content areas and the methods of general psychology are, by definition, relevant to a large number of social problems. Community psychology need only draw on this diverse background of existing information to help alleviate the problems: When the "therapy" of community psychology becomes job-training, it is also educational psychology, when it becomes preschool programs, it is cognitive-developmental psychology, when it becomes community organization, it is social psychology, when it becomes a personal consultant to people it is clinical psychology, and so on. There is virtually no area of human behavior that cannot be claimed by the community psychologist as a legitimate community mental health activity.

Community mental health, so defined, is seen by some as a humanitarian development and the actualization of egalitarian values. Within universities, such programs are seen as a move toward relevance and toward fulfilling new found social and community responsibilities. It is seen as humanitarian to help people deal with problems that are destroying their potential for happiness. It is also considered egalitarian to make professional mental health services, formerly restricted to the wealthy, available to large numbers of people. Community mental health is so presented by the professionals, who stand ready to fill this expanded concept of mental health and who of course will be its principal financial beneficiaries. Community psychology can be included within the scope of the movement.

What are the benefits and costs to society? Are there dangers which have been overlooked by the new perspective of the mental health movement?

The psychotherapeutic state: A hidden danger

There is a hidden issue of paramount importance, but one which has not surfaced in an articulate way. If community psychology becomes an extension of the political arm of the government in the name of humanitarian goals and egalitarian values, it will be a grand deception which is contrary to the interests of the people and also to the values it claims to serve. Again, the issue of exercising control over others by mental health professionals and the value of so doing needs to be examined. This time the issue has implications for those academic institutions which are establishing community-psychology training programs and are consciously sheltering the community mental health movement.

The dimensions of the hidden danger can be seen in the concept of the "therapeutic state" in which the mental health movement serves the political aims of the government. In Russia, psychiatric hospitalization has been used as a means of controlling and regulating troublesome intellectuals.[1] Yet, the Soviets are not alone in this abuse of psychiatry. In the United States, a similar move toward the therapeutic state can be found in the acceptance by the government of the mental health ideology of providing mental health services for low-income groups who, by the definition of community mental health, need such services.

PSYCHO-ADAPTATION OF THE POOR. According to the community psychologist Robert Reiff, the poor do not want mental health services; they see them as irrelevant to their needs.[2] The mental health movement is solidly built upon middle-class values. It is staffed by white middle-class professionals, and armed with concepts in which a person is seen as a victim of his own self, an intrapsychic view. Mental health is self-actualization. But the lower classes see themselves as victims of circumstances, and thus they do not see mental health as being relevant. For them, the causes are seen as completely external and the social forces and institutions are what should be changed.

The mental health solution, places blame on the poor, not on inadequate institutions. The alternative to defining the poor as inferior people in need of critical attention is the recognition of institutional failure. That failure cries out for critical attention. But, institutional forces are never geared to critical self-analysis. In fact, it is the alienation of the lower-class person from the institutional world that defined his need for professional services in the first place.

These institutional aspects of society provide the funds, not to change themselves, but to modify those defined as the problem. If the poor can be diagnosed as sick, then they are the problem. In that sense, the mental health expert has offered to cure the afflicted and diverted attention from institutional factors. The mental health movement would impose on the poor a treatment and ethic they neither wanted nor asked for, but that they, the professionals, are prepared to give. The community mental health movement is a majority decision to deal with the poor through a mental health ideology, and it is in this respect community psychology as a part of the movement becomes the handmaiden of the state.

A central issue is the control over resources. Consider police work. It is conceivable that psychology could have some useful applications in the area of police-community relations and police-citizen interaction. Public awareness and willingness to support police functions are at a high level; but, the principal money to support research is administered by the justice department and has frequently been used to buy more sophisticated weaponry. Psychologists may expect to receive money as long as their projects support the police in their police work. The possible critical analysis is controlled by the police; the institutional forces operate to help the majority assimilate the misfits.

Psychology, and the social sciences in general, are developing understandings which can be used for the effective control of human behavior. Given access to children through the schools and to selected populations through community programs, significant manipulation of the behavior, emotions, and attitudes of people can be attempted. Basic research now makes that possible. Community psychologists and the mental health movement stand ready to serve the community as social change agents for institutionalized forms of power. Poverty, alienation, lack of self-identity, and so on, will become the focal point of the mental health expert as he promises to reclaim for majority society those large segments of nonconformists and misfits whose very existence defines a social problem.

THE NEW DEFENSE CONTRACTS. Community psychology programs, as part of our university graduate training programs, will be (and are being) called upon to play a part in the new mental health ideology. The assumption of this role by our universities should be considered as potentially dangerous as their acceptance of defense contracts for developing sophisticated tools of war. These tools, of course, can be conceptual rather than material, such as nuclear fusion was in one case, and as reinforcement or brain processes may become now.

If the university accepts its assigned role for community psychology within the current mental health movement, it will take one further step along the road toward becoming an arm for government control. For a variety of reasons, the university is not now *apolitical*, but some important distinctions have been blurred. Some demands for institutional activity, such as the opposition to the Vietnam war, are inconsistent with established power and rejected as political and inappropriate, while others, such as the assigned role of community psychology in the mental health movement, are consistent and accepted as nonpolitical and appropriate.

Unfortunately, the issue has not been dealt with in a straightforward way. Should we recognize the apolitical posture of our universities as a myth and then fight over what aims they are to serve? Or, should we try to redefine what is an appropriate role for the university?

Appropriate community psychology

It is possible to envision a community psychology program in an academic setting which is appropriate. Such a program would be free to serve an unrestrained critical function. This mythical program would not, however, conveniently fit into the current mental health movement or even be consistent with much of contemporary psychology.

As an academic program, what form would community psychology take within an academic institution? It would be devoted to the scientific study and understanding of the psychological aspects of community problems, for example, how to conceptualize ghetto life. Such a program has been called for by a black psychologist who has pointed out the need to study such things as the sociopolitical arrangements which determine the behavior of those who differ from white norms.[3] Research conducted by an establishment-based psychology

173

against the poor must give way to research investigating those processes and institutions which lock the poor into poverty.

There are some research programs of this type, most of which have been funded by research agencies of the federal government.[4] These efforts, however, are relatively few. They are small and inconsequential compared with the size and scope of the mental health movement. It is the mental health movement itself which is the principal danger. This movement derives its strength from the professional aspirations which promote it and from the service agencies of the government which buy it. Both are accumulating institutionalized power that acts in its own self-interest rather than in the interests of those they claim to serve.

To move in an appropriate direction would have many implications for the institutional milieu. For example, white middle-class psychologists function in ways which reflect their own background, training, and experience. The use of middle-class concepts and theories necessarily overlooks those norms that are peculiar to disadvantaged ethnic and minority groups. It is impossible for contemporary psychology to conduct appropriate community psychology without first seeing how current institutionalized policies sustain and contribute to this incapacity.

The issue is not an academic one, because psychology has within its power the capacity to effect institutional changes which could make community psychology a viable science. Consider admission to graduate school. Only a small percentage of all Ph.D. psychologists are black among a national population that includes about 11 percent. The population that represents the target for community psychology may be 50 percent or more black. But, what would be the consequence of a greater percentage of black psychologists?

Many of the blacks accepted could be expected to add a different perspective and new diversity to community psychology programs. However, these same individuals, if they came from low socio-economic backgrounds, would be as out of place in a private clinic consulting on the identity crisis of a socialite, as the traditional clinical psychologist is now out of place trying to consult with a sixteen-year-old ghetto black who is an armed-robbery parolee and who came from a fatherless home with eight siblings. The research and service aspects of clinical psychology would have to shift to accommodate the new diversity added to the training program. But academics enjoy their artificial world and they have built it to protect their own image.

Research would also change. Allotments of space in professional journals would have to be realigned. So would the relative positions of power and influence within academic departments. In short, psychology would become a somewhat different discipline.

In the context just presented, the establishment of an appropriate community psychology would also have to reflect a political movement within psychology. The power structure within the field of psychology would be at stake. However, if the appropriate function of an academic department is to explore community questions to their logical limit, and also to be critical of ideas and concepts, and finally to investigate on an unrestricted front, then the current emergence of community psychology would be healthy. Its promises for accomplishment, of course, would be much more modest than those of the mental health movement, but such a difference always lies between inquiry and proselytizing. Can psychology honestly extend itself to the community without internal institutional change, or can it exclude the community and yet honestly present itself as psychology?

AS PROFESSIONAL SERVICE. Psychology is a profession as well as a science. The addition of an appropriate academic community psychology program would have applied consequences. The new graduates who left such a university program, similar to many Ph.D.s in clinical psychology, would take service jobs in the community. If they continued in the professional role of serving the needs of their clients, whether or not they corresponded with the aims of the mental health movement, their service function would parallel the academic role in the sense that institutional change would be promoted rather than a further effort to control deviant behavior through a mental health ideology.

It should be noted that the American Psychology Association, in a statement of keen awareness, issued a position paper on what should be the structure of community mental health centers.[5] This statement asserted that if the Community Mental Health Centers were to become effective community agents, community representatives must be actively involved in setting goals and determining basic policy. Any professional worker who followed the APA-recommended policy as to his proper role would be working for, and therefore be *accountable* to, the community.

Such accountability, however, has further internal consequences for psychology. A black psychologist who has rejected the framework of white-dominated psychology which emphasizes internal psychological processes and holds himself (as a professional) accountable to a clientele who consider external factors as responsible for their condition, will engage in very different activities. Consider the use of psychological tests. These instruments serve an essentially conservative function in society of finding people who fit preexisting opportunities, and by definition, exclude societal misfits from opportunity.

In more concrete terms, exposure to an inner-city school program will ensure inferior educational experiences, low test scores, and therefore exclusion from jobs and higher education; this, in turn, ensures further confinement to the inner-city school. We have come full circle, not to mention the toll of frustration and failure, of lost hope, and ultimately anger.

It is a strange paradox, because tests are held up as the accepted way to be fair and to show that nondiscriminatory practices are followed. Programs of admission to jobs or educational programs on a quota or on an opportunities program basis have not been supported either conceptually or with the financial support necessary to make them workable. But, it must be realized that psychologists play an important role in maintaining testing and admission procedures. Commercial tests turn large profits and provide sizable amounts of money for the employment of psychologists and for paid advertising which helps to support journals and professional meetings. There is little money for those forces which fail to support or which would be in opposition to the conservative function served by tests and by the psychologists hired to maintain the psychometric tradition.

The effective community psychologist, in practice, if he functioned in an appropriate way, would come into conflict with other psychologists and produce tension within the existing structure of psychology. Again, the disclaimer should be made that such psychologists would not solve the problems of the poor or the misfit; they would help to remove the problems from the mental health context and oppose the therapeutic state.

An appropriate community psychology program would require institutional change at many levels. It should be clearly and forcefully noted, however, that such a community psychology program is neither antiscientific or antiintellectual. At no time has the value of psychometric instruments been questioned. They are necessary and important tools. Measuring instruments are necessary for any science to further scientific understanding. In the illustration used, the instruments are not serving scientific purposes, they are serving the purposes of established and strong vested interests. These interests, in turn, control many of the directions psychology may take as a discipline; change is not in their interest nor is the open development of forces which question the humanitarian aims and egalitarian values used to justify their position.

A POINT OF CONFUSION. Many psychologists who support academic freedom have reservations about whether community psychology, as just described, is appropriate. The confusion arises over the failure to make a distinction between what is a political struggle *within* psychology, and the relation of the university or profession to the state. In one of its uses, "political" refers to the relationship of the state toward institutions, or institutions toward their members. In this context, an apolitical institution is not the ideological servant of the state, or the individual of the institution. *This distinction is the essence of academic freedom* and it must be maintained if community psychology is to avoid furthering the establishment of the therapeutic state and preserve its function of critical inquiry.

In another of its uses, "political" refers to the relation of members toward their institutions, such as the university or professional associations to which they belong. At this level, political activity is an appropriate process which serves as a mechanism for internal change. However, as we have seen, the established forces within psychology are protecting a vested interest which is dependent upon justifying a role the institutions may serve in the mental health movement as an ideological agent

178

of the state. It is not, therefore, surprising that these individuals have opposed the type of community psychology proposed here. But, in so doing, they also have managed to mistake appropriate internal resistance against their role as "political" activity which threatens the university. The victim of this confusion has been the critical function of the university and profession. *It is the position of the university and profession with respect to the state which is the critical relationship for determining appropriate from inappropriate activity.* Clinical psychology as a principal academic home of the community mental health movement and of community psychology is in a unique position to help resolve and clarify these important issues.

Dangers from without

There are very real external dangers to academic freedom even if the internal dangers are avoided and an active but appropriate community psychology program is established. At the level of scientific understanding, there is the danger of a withdrawal from the university of the funds which are needed to support the faculty and their research. General reductions in appropriations reduce the critical functioning of a university because fixed operating costs then consume, in the limiting case, all of the money available. Research support would then be totally dependent upon sources external to the university and thus subject to external control. As examples, other dangers include direct intervention by the state legislature into the university in such forms as the reevaluation of tenure, loss of administrative control, and line item control over the budgets.

At the professional service level, the operation of community mental health centers depends upon a professional staff provided for by government money. Thus, without institutional changes, the

179

service aspect of community psychology cannot really ever be accountable to the community, but only to the state director of mental health, *a political appointee*.

An appropriate research or service function could result in a loss of academic and professional freedom. These issues are very real. Majority society, at this point in time, does not want effective critics, and apparently cannot find sufficient reasons to support them. There is not an objection to critical inquiry in principle, but just to the consequences. It is the fear of these dangers from without that marshalls some forces within the university to purge themselves of the faculty and activities which displease the institutionalized power of the mental health movement. The rationale for the purge is that the offensive activities are political, and thus have no place in a university.

The dilemma is multileveled. In one sense it is like being offered a choice of either being shot or hanged and then being abused for showing insufficient appreciation for the choice offered. If the university continues its trend toward becoming an arm for that part of the government which has accepted the mental health ideology, it does violence to self-proclaimed academic values; but, if it moves toward an appropriate stand, equal damage may well be done by the wrath from without which follows. No one who has the decisions on his shoulders has been particularly appreciative of the choice offered, nor do they seem to have an easy out.

Of course it can, and perhaps should, be questioned whether an academic freedom and critical function which can so easily be impaled on the horns of this dilemma is a reality at all, or only a myth.

None of the options is attractive. There are two honest and one dishonest, but perhaps expedient, alternatives: (a) The university could openly become an agent for the mental health ideology in exchange for money and government support. It is an honest choice, but one that would entail a considerable change in proclaimed self-identity; (b) the other honest alternative is to reestablish an institution which is free to serve a critical function and to maintain the integrity of academic freedom, but at a risk of loss of financial support. This alternative is based on the premise that there is necessarily an incompatible relationship between an academic institution and the professional services it renders for the government; (c) the expedient alternative is the mental health movement option of supporting a community psychology program acceptable to the government while denying that the university is an arm of the governmental and professional power of the mental health movement.

Relevance

Community psychology has partially achieved its current rapid growth in popularity because it can present itself to all sides as an appropriate solution and as a move toward relevance. It is a remarkable accomplishment, which can be accounted for only by the ambiguity of the definition of community mental health.

For the state, relevance is the first alternative. The university is to serve society. For community psychology, it is to adapt the misfits and deviants to majority society, even against their wishes, without due process, and, adding insult to injury, in the name of humanitarian values provided by the mental health movement. This would be a new university serving the ends of majority society.

For the majority of students, relevance in a university includes such things as a community psychology program, but not in the first sense. They want the university to serve a critical function, even of government and of majority society. These students are not yet so cynical as to believe that the university is indistinguishable from the other institutions of the military-industrial complex. It remains to be seen if this judgment is too generous. For some, however, the university is seen as an entrenched political institution and the struggle for relevance in the university is no different from the struggle for political control of all of our institutions toward a redistribution of power.

Among faculty and administrators there are a few purists, who want the second option but devoid of a program like community psychology. It is the ivory tower. Perhaps the issue is not so much academic freedom as much as it is academic isolation. This is a position which is fading because there are few new supporters. My own view is that it is a quaint position, charming for older scholars, appropriate for a time past, but no longer a viable alternative. Principally because science has become so complex and so expensive that an individual scientist can no longer be philosophically isolated from political commerce with institutional forces, such as his university and his professional organizations.

The majority of faculty and administrators live in the make-believe world of the third alternative; doing the first while claiming the second. The process of rationalizing the contradiction is a consuming obsession which becomes more demanding with each new stress. It is a tremendous burden which is crushing the university but which provides temporary relief by shifting attention away from the basic horns of the dilemma. The strategy has, for now, succeeded in confusing the argument to the point where the conflict between these options is no longer central.

The choice

Universities are not facing the larger issue, nor

is psychology facing the specific case provided by community psychology. The important issues have been obscured and we, as professional psychologists, are carried forward by our own momentum and economic self-interest. The ultimate resolution is a collective one, and heavy responsibility rests on our collective organizations, such as professional societies and university senates. But, collective progress must come from individual initiative and personal resolve to undertake the appropriate internal political reform to achieve an appropriate external position and secure an unencumbered critical function. Community psychology is an ideal focal point with which to clear our heads.

Perhaps my own views are already obvious, but they should be made explicit if we are to be on with the debate. We need community psychology programs which are not part of the mental health ideology. Understanding human behavior is beyond the ivory tower; it must include the real world. To serve this larger critical function, we must make institutional changes; one specific example is black admissions and all the professional consequences and disruptions of our status quo which such a change entails. Not the least of which will be a confrontation with the state. An adversary relationship with the government and even majority society is an unpleasant thought and probably economically suicidal. But that confrontation is coming on many levels, as man is slowly coming to the awakening that he must gain control over his life or face institutionalized control from which there is no escape and no sense of self. With careful work, the confrontation can be conceptual and the revolution cultural. Can a university afford to be anything other than on the side of truth and courage? Let us develop an appropriate community psychology rather than allow it to devolve further as an element of the therapeutic state.

13

action
for
mental
health

One's perspective of madness depends on what events are defined as relevant and the context in which they are placed. The perspective presented in this book must be seen as an invented interpretation imposed on the domain of madness. Now that this perspective has been presented, it is necessary to explore the implications it provides for the future. It is not necessary for the reader to share the views presented in this book or to be convinced that the solutions offered are the most relevant or important ones. But, if the perspectives provided are to be rejected, they must be rejected with some justification and in light of possible alternatives. The intent has been to define dimensions relevant to the problem of madness which either must be acknowledged and then dealt with, or excluded on some other grounds as irrelevant.

Practical versus scientific perspectives

Clearly there is a fundamental and radical difference in the perspective of madness provided by the applied and scientific viewpoint. The material on clinical formulation and decisions seems to suggest almost no direct guidelines for what the practicing clinician can or should do now—today—when confronted with such human problems.

Such a discrepancy between science and practice will always exist no matter how or at what time one views it. Decisions always must be made on what seem to be the most relevant grounds. At times the growth in a basic science permits the applied practitioner to proceed to his task with greater dispatch and efficiency than at other times. Growth in basic scientific information causes major upheavals in the social order and in so doing *redefines* the practical problems and practical implications to be faced. In the field of psychopathology, present information is such that the *fundamental nature of the mental health movement needs to be reexamined.* The prospects for the future seem sufficiently clear to indicate the direction of change that is needed. The practical problems as they are currently defined will not be solved by a science of human behavior, but will rather be given a *redefinition* in terms of the future. The necessary action for mental health lies in a fundamental upheaval of the current mental health movement in order for it to become compatible with the prospect provided by the biological and social sciences.

THE SHIFTING FOCUS. The scientific perspective, which can include both dynamic and behavioral concepts, will open new possibilities for handling people. If we follow this perspective through to its logical consequences, we must start to answer the question of who is to be modified and in what way. These are ethical and moral questions having to do with arriving at a definition of suitable behavior for society. The point, and it is a simple one, is that the behavioral sciences and the biological sciences will provide techniques for conceptualizing behavior which will permit *behavior* to be controlled, to be modified, and to be dealt with at a practical level. The important question is what behavior is to be desired or tolerated and what behavior is to be eliminated. We are pointing here to the fundamental question of the amount of variability in behavior that society will permit and the conditions and the circumstances under which society will undertake to modify the behavior that its members show.

The perspective afforded by science does not tell us what we should do, but rather what can be done. On the other hand, the current mental health propaganda pretends that science has determined what adjustment and normality are. The primary problem is not mental illness as currently iden- tified, but how to live with a science of human behavior. This must be faced anew, rather than on traditional medical grounds and the opinion of mental health experts. Appropriate behavior is a relative concept which must be seen in the context of the social values of the time.

The current mental health movement is set up to eradicate an illness—such as madness—and put in its place health, such as adjustment. This approach implies an article of faith, namely that science will be able to discover what adjustment or happiness is, and provide techniques to instill it. Nothing could be less realistic. The scientific perspective does *not* include values; it does not include information about how man should live with man. The scientific perspective will provide increasingly sophisticated ways of viewing human behavior and the possibility for increased control over behavior. Just as man has altered his environment to suit his needs, so too will he develop the technology to deal with his fellow man. The question then becomes one of how to live with this information, not one of waiting for science to deliver some utopia. If we wait for the utopia, we will find ourselves confronted with a technology with which we are not prepared to live.

AN OPEN AND PUBLIC SOCIETY. We have claimed that man is now in the position to begin development of a science of human behavior. Such a development implies behavior control. A further consequence is a deepening conflict between science and the current practices which we have referred to as the mental health movement. The conflict concerns current practices that are inconsistent and misrepresent scientific information. The conflict is fundamental and will have many far-reaching effects.

One of these effects should be the elimination of the role of the mental health expert and a requirement for an open and public definition of the purposes and ends for which behavior control may be used. A new expert will emerge at the applied level to implement these actions. The decision, however, as to what situations and toward what ends these implementations may take place must, in a constitutional democracy, be removed from the opinion of the expert. This will be necessary because the bases for these decisions are not inherent in the technology nor in the science. Currently the mental health expert has claimed these prerogatives and has obtained legislative right for his claim to exercise them. The claim is false by current standards of science and is contrary to the values of an open and free society.

It should be made explicitly clear that this is *not* an argument against treatment, but rather the context under which it is done. There are many problems of living in modern society and the structure of modern society will require the collective acceptance of social responsibility for helping individual people who have these problems. However, in a democratic society, the intrusions of the institutional forces into the lives of others must be under legislative and constitutional restrictions. The state will have to provide employees for this function, but, as agents of the state, the grounds for their activity must be open and public.

Government control is a key issue. In the United States, the mental health movement provides an indirect means for such control through the therapeutic state. The mental health professional is coming forth as the new inquisitor and undermining the values of an open and public society. The mental health professional does have an important applied role to play, but we must be explicit about this role. It must be rendered commensurate with the scientific perspective and the excess functions that the mental health expert now fills must be removed from his prerogative and returned to the public domain.

SCIENCE AND HUMANISM. Our dynamic approaches to personality have attempted to capture the ongoing, vivid and personal experiences of living: the sometimes happy and the sometimes sad experiences out of which we ourselves, and our ambitions, desires, and troubles are founded, satisfied, frustrated, or changed. From a naturalistic standpoint, the capacity to have such feelings and emotions seems so uniquely human and seems to define what we mean by happiness or unhappiness, and madness or sanity. However, it is this dynamic view which has been rejected, but only to the extent that it has been correlated with the role of the mental health expert, the concept of mental illness, and the mental health movement as we now know it. It is important to be clear on the point that it is

189

only the practical applied role which has been challenged. Dynamic as well as behavioral concepts comprise the scientific perspective.

The scientific perspective is not antihumanistic. Tenderness, love, and other such experiences are undoubtedly important aspects of human behavior. Man will continue to study himself in order to better understand what tenderness, or love, or identity means. But when we know this—and the prospects are emerging—there will then be the practical implications of this information being used in ways incompatible with the values we hold. Science cannot sell love, or tenderness, or identity—only insofar as the products of increased knowledge of man as a biological and social organism can be put in service toward particular values. Humanistic accomplishments are to be found in these values, not in holding onto the role of the mental health expert because he or she claims to use humanistic terms. The time has come to face the issue of behavior control, and it must be placed in the open and public realm.

ASSUMPTIONS OF THE REDEFINITION. The basic assertions made in the redefinition can be listed as a reference point for proposing specific courses of action:

(1) Mental health and illness should be abandoned as an absolute state or condition of the organism for which science will provide the definition.

(2) The behavioral sciences will provide techniques for the modification of behavior. But the principal new task is to determine the limits of application of these techniques and the direction and goals toward which they are to be applied.

(3) The mental health movement at the applied level needs to be reevaluated, replacing the role of the mental health expert with a workable alternative for aiding individuals who are having difficulties.

(4) At a conceptual level, the type of human

190

problems the dynamic alternative has attempted to deal with and the scientific rigor of the behavioral alternative, need to be brought into closer working relationship in order to provide useful knowledge toward the construction of a technology applicable to human problems.

These assertions essentially demand that we face the implications of lifting the concept of madness from the context of illness and medicine to a nonmedical context of problems of living. If we do this, the implications concerning both how the mental health movement should be managed and the role and responsibility of various parties toward the psychiatric patient are far-reaching. By treating madness as a problem of living in all its social and ethical aspects, we will directly face problems of values that are otherwise hidden. To bring these issues into the open raises new questions concerning the manpower and the logistics of madness in our contemporary society.

Positive steps of action

MANPOWER—A BROADER BASE. One of the conclusions of psychologist William Schofield was that the service psychotherapists are providing is friendship for a price.[1] He concludes that the "talking" cure of psychotherapy has not led to the alleviation of the mental health problem, but it has helped people through the friendship provided by therapists. Yet there is an insufficient supply of therapists to provide that necessary friendship.

Given the ratio of one person in ten who will be hospitalized and the added millions the Joint Commission said needed professional help because of problems in living, and given the efforts of psychologists and psychiatrists to keep the mental health profession closed, the present lack of manpower is guaranteed to continue. The mental health experts, via union and guild characteristics, have established themselves as the only ones entitled and sufficiently trained to carry out the delicate treatment of psychotherapy. There is thus a small group of professional people whose friendship may be purchased by those affluent enough to afford it.

A more damaging fact, however, than the reduction of psychotherapy to the mere purchase of friendship, is that most psychiatrists and clinical psychologists are not using their special training. The psychiatrist is first of all trained in medicine and has extensive knowledge about the body as a biological system. The clinical psychologist has extensive training in the social and behavioral sciences and knowledge of human behavior in its social settings. The psychologist receives a Ph.D. degree which includes training in research; his special skills enable him to plan experiments which can bear upon theoretical questions and to process and handle data in a way which will provide meaningful answers. When the psychiatrist or the psychologist practices the talking cure of psychotherapy, he utilizes virtually none of his special training. Much of a psychiatrist's medical training is irrelevant to the work and responsibility assumed in the mental health profession. [2] The point, simply made, is that the training that psychologists and psychiatrists receive is *irrelevant* to what they are currently doing as mental health experts.

The implication of the structure of the current mental health field is that our federal government, by training grants and federal resources, and our state governments, by the support of graduate departments and medical schools, are turning out highly specialized people who do not use the skills for which they are trained, and who serve no generally useful purpose to the society. Rather they provide friendship which may be purchased by an affluent few. Further, it is our conclusion that the service they are selling has no scientific justification; little proof exists for its usefulness.

If one takes seriously the recommendations of the Joint Commission, that the most important need is for more verifiable knowledge and information, these highly trained experts should be contributing to the enterprise for which they are uniquely fitted by training, and not to the one which exploits public resources to provide an unproven product for a select group of the general population.

The solution seems to require a broader base for the mental health movement. If, in fact, clinical psychologists and psychiatrists are not using the skills they are especially trained for, then other people should be recruited who are capable of assuming much of the responsibility that the professional now carries. If one further grants that the problem is primarily a nonmedical problem, then people other than clinical psychologists and psychiatrists *should* be involved, such as happily married couples, college students, social workers, educators, and any other persons who are familiar with the problem, successful, and warm. Once the concept of mental illness has been changed to one of disordered behavior in a social context, there is a wave of qualified manpower that can be called upon to bear the brunt of handling and processing the people society will single out for special attention and friendship because of problems of living.

Part of the solution that seems to be called for is a return to moral treatment. This term is based on the concept of setting the patient a good example and emphasizing an atmosphere of kindness and good advice. It was brought to this country by the Quakers. It does not pretend to provide scientific information or the gifts of research, but reflects the current social wisdom. The person practicing moral therapy is to be a person who is a sensitive observer

193

of situations and circumstances and who can provide helpful suggestions about problems of living. There are many successful people who have managed their lives efficiently and effectively, and who are recognized for it by their peers. They can provide friendship.

Unabashed and imbued with personal values representative of those in society in general, these people can help others who are in need of friendship and who are having problems in living. They can help these people, look at the ways in which they are leading their lives (i.e., their behavior) in terms of what they are doing, what other people are doing, and what alternatives are open. At this level one simply deals with the way a person is behaving and what he says he feels. It is public and open. The focus is on the behavior, unobscured by mystical concepts such as postpartem depression, anal-erotic, obsessive symptoms, oedipal complex, ataxic mobility of the psychic energy, deepening of interests, strengthening of ego identity, and so on. The host of processes, concepts, and structures within the personality are left in the hands of a scientific perspective until they can be empirically grounded, experimentally tested, and proved worthy of being marketed.

If this is done, if madness is confronted at the level of the values that society and people wish to maintain, at the level of actual behavior, then as the new information becomes available providing a more sophisticated view of the human organism, we will be better prepared to know what we want to do with this information. *As it now stands such new information threatens the current justification for professional practice and the mental health expert stands in opposition to new knowledge and change.*

Implicit in the approach proposed is that both professional and nonprofessional mental health workers occupy salaried positions. The number of treatment hours available could be expanded at no greater cost by providing less expensive, non-professional salaried positions through which concerned and dedicated people can bring their own personal experience and effective past behaviors to provide influence, models, assurance, and direct suggestions to people who are having difficulty with their lives. It is not the role of our medical and graduate schools to train people to establish a closed society to sell such friendship to a few people.

The psychiatrist and the clinical psychologist with their special training are the ones on whom the burden must fall of providing the verifiable information called for by the Joint Commission on Mental Illness and Health. There is room for two kinds of research, and these people can make two very different but equally important contributions. On the one hand we have the need for pure research which provides the general stock of knowledge on which the progress of the future is always built. This research can be as far removed from the mental health field as paired associate learning of nonsense syllables, salivary conditioning of the dog, or biochemical processes in the body. On the other hand, many individuals with research talent cannot turn their backs on the problems and sufferings of their fellow man even for the moment. For these individuals there are opportunities for applied research. The task of transforming the abstract theoretical information of a science perspective into a workable technology requires people sophisticated both in scientific information and in the practical aspects of madness.

The applied research individual would remain close to patients but carry out an experimental and critical function; it would not be a professional effort which required the pretensions of special knowledge. This person should also be in a salaried position working as a scientist to bring the information of the biological and social sciences to bear on man and his social order. It is at this level that the moral dilemma exists. At this level we must focus on the behavior of people and the conditions under which we are willing to attempt to effect changes toward solving human problems. My argument is that it is fundamentally wrong and a misconception about the role of science in society to expect that science will specify how this information is to be used. The most important task is a reshaping of the mental health movement.

Abolishing the professional guild

I do not wish to see psychiatrists or clinical psychologists leave the applied field of mental health. I do not wish to see them stop talking or working with patients. It is unlikely that a more sophisticated and more powerful view of human behavior can ever be achieved without continuing to look and listen to man himself. In reflecting on my own career as a clinical psychologist, it seems that when I have been most effective I have responded to my patients as an individual concerned about their behavior and helping them behave in ways that had better consequences for them and which made them feel better. My dynamic notions of personality, if anything, got in the way of what I could do for them as a sensible and concerned individual. A case history of my personal experience, of course, does not prove any point. I am merely adding my personal conviction to what seems to be the logical conclusion of prohibiting the sale of a product that has failed to meet even the minimum standards of science. Notice, I am not against this service being provided by society. There is a demand and a market for friendship. I am objecting to its being sold as science, *and* to its being offered by a select group of people who remain select *by virtue of training which they do not use.* The net effect of this process is to hinder the solution of a critical problem in two ways: first, by insuring an insufficient supply of therapists, and second, by hiding the fundamental questions of values that must be answered in order to prepare for the dilemma of living with a science of human behavior.

In this context, the mental health movement in its current form is detrimental to the best interests of society. Clinical psychologists and psychiatrists with their special organizations are protecting vested interests which are at the source of the problem. The responsible action will be to abolish the guilds that perpetuate the contemporary view of madness. The answer is to open the door to an echelon of manpower willing and capable of meeting the pressures of providing others with help in problems of living while freeing the professional manpower for pure and applied research. The professionals themselves need to lower the restrictive barriers they have constructed for economic protection or have it done for them. One course of action would be to establish a stepladder of mental health workers ranging from specialists through professionals, paraprofessionals, technicians, assistants, and aides on which people would be free to climb in status, either through experience on the job, formal training or a combination of both. The importance of degrees would be reduced while the capacity to do a job would be emphasized. The open-ended spectrum would attract qualified workers at all levels and the social resources mobilized for helping people with problems, but stripped of the medical context and the guild structure which insures both an inadequate and inappropriate response.

THE BOULDER MODEL. Many clinical psychology programs still operate under the Boulder model of a "scientist-professional." This is a view of a psychologist as a person who has carried out scholarly research for his Ph.D. but who works as a professional in an applied setting, bringing to the setting the critical function of the scholar. The model has been a complete failure.

Why has the model failed? For one reason, the job market does not support a "scientist-professional" type of person. The number of psychologists has increased by over 100 percent in the last decade. These individuals have taken jobs which pay for service functions and reward individuals for fitting into the mental health system. Economic position is secured by mental health expansion into new areas, achievement of health insurance payments, and the formation of organizations and associations to lobby for favorable standing with legislative support. With this role there has been a loss of capacity for the critical function for which the Ph.D. is trained.

A further reason why the scientist-professional has failed has been for a lack of individuals who fit the description. Many degree candidates in clinical psychology have suffered through the research requirements in order to have access to a responsible helping position. The opening of a spectrum of mental health jobs short of the Ph.D. would give this person a direct route to his goals rather than through a graduate program in which most of his specialized training is wasted. Those left to receive the research training would have an appropriate place in the field consistent with their interests and training.

Change has been slow to come because academic departments have been all too willing to train people in the scientist-professional model. This training task floated academic psychology to positions of relative power and size within our universities. To maintain that position, scientific psychology must embrace the professional, who now, to maintain his own position, has goals contrary to those of academia. The vision of a scientist-professional combined in one person did not solve the basic incompatibility in the past and will not do so now. The incompatibility rests upon the nature of the mental health movement and the effort of academic departments to serve both critical and service functions; the contradiction will be resolved only by effecting institutional changes, especially in the mental health movement.

COMMUNITY PSYCHOLOGY. The future growth potential of psychology is now in the extension of the role of the mental health expert into the arena of community mental health. The temptation for Ph.D. programs will be to accept a part of this movement on the terms offered by the mental health movement; the result will be a further loss of critical function and a further politicizing of the university. In contrast, *appropriate* extensions into community psychology will first entail a political struggle within psychology to establish a community psychology that is not part of the therapeutic state and which perseveres in critical inquiry. The place of an academic program is to encourage free spirits and critical functions. The professional worker, to function in the same way, must be accountable to those he seeks to represent. Thus, there is a role for the psychologist in the community, but not on the terms provided by social psychiatry and the current mental health movement.

REDUCING THE DEMAND. Related to the supply problem is the large demand for mental health services. At least part of the problem is the present *definition* of what constitutes mental illness. Currently this includes the interpretation of sundry social problems as manifestations of mental illness, proposals for yearly mental health check-ups, and the equation of subjective happiness with mental health. In this latter vein, failure to enjoy one's role in life as student, mother, mechanic, professor, or what have you, is taken as a sign of lack of adjustment. Subjective happiness and a purpose in life have become a human right to be implemented by professional psychiatric and psychological groups. Simply to make the problem smaller by a redefinition of mental illness and the appropriate role of the mental health expert is neither callous nor short-sighted.

I am not against happiness nor a sense of purpose and self-satisfaction with one's role in life; nor indeed, even against the idea as seen as a human right. But these aspects of living are best viewed in the context of social problems with the realm of action falling to education, political organizations and structures, economic institutions, and so on—not health. In part, the individuals involved in such a crisis need to be seen as persons in need of simple friendship. The mental health context, however, is not the appropriate one for giving friendship. Mental health has been oversold as to what problems are to be defined and therefore dealt with by the mental health movement. The demand will be smaller if we will redefine problems into more appropriate categories; for example, to treat the problems of the poor more as an economic question or one of political ideology, and less as mental inadequacy. It is not that, psychologically, the poor lack a sense of the future as much as they lack a real future.

INVOLUNTARY HOSPITALIZATION. Szasz has argued, as is argued here, that a person must be held responsible for his behavior. To hold him responsible offers him the opportunity to gain self-respect. Mental illness cannot be a mitigating condition. This way, society will act collectively against members who deviate from its norms on the basis of their behavior. In our society, a criminal cannot be convicted until found guilty of an unlawful act. It follows that a person must have the right to behave deviantly before he can be committed for his problems of living. It is incumbent on the social order to make

200

clear that involuntary commitment is an act of one's fellow man seeking to control certain behavior. In a democratic society, such control cannot be exercised lightly, for it then becomes dictatorial. Such an open system does not need to be *non-humanitarian*. In theory, we decide where to place our criminals by taking into account the kinds of institutions available and the particular individual in question. The same may be true of involuntary hospitalization where the placement and the actions taken are geared to the needs of the individual in question, but within the context of a public and open system of moral philosophy and values.

Such an approach would require that the psychiatrist and the clinical psychologist give up their roles as experts in judging the mental health of individuals brought before the court. The question of primary concern is what the person has done, the circumstances that the person finds himself in, and whether, in its collective fashion, society is willing to give instruments to some of its agents to force an alternative on the individual. The charge of madness must always be open and public and the criteria, as much as possible, placed within the context of a *nonmedical* value system. This does not mean, of course, the psychiatrist or the clinical psychologist would never testify in court; indeed, their opinions might at one time or another be valuable in assisting the court to make a disposition (not determination) of an individual case.

ELIMINATING THE BEHAVIORAL-DYNAMIC CONTROVERSY. At the level of scientific inquiry, there is no conflict between the dynamic and the behavioral. They are different levels of explanation and make different assumptions about how to approach the task of understanding human behavior. Both must use the same rules for evaluating their concepts. The extent to which either or both will produce useful concepts is an empirical question. The ultimate verification is the empirically demonstrated practical implications of a resulting technology.

This book has implied that as the dynamic type of concepts become verified, they will be modified and in the process will become similar in form to the behavioral view. Problems of clinical formulation and decision will be handled by a technology oriented toward behavior control. Such an integration can take place only when the various professional groups contribute toward obtaining verifiable knowledge and toward its application, with the ends determined on other grounds. This will not be easy to achieve within the social realities of the profession and the present professional framework.

In another sense, the behavioral-dynamic controversy is not reconcilable. At the applied level is the belief that dynamic concepts will yield a view that may appropriately be called mental health. This represents faith in the dynamic assumptions about personality which justifies a professional guild. At the level of this basic assumption, there is no escape from the current controversy.

Scientific responsibility and mental health

It would be a mistake if this book, without qualification, cast the mental health movement, professional practices, and the commercially marketed dynamic viewpoint as the villain, and cast the scientific community and its practices and viewpoints as the hero. Such melodramatic identifications were useful to sharpen the distinctions in much of the preceding material between abuses and virtues but was, of necessity, achieved only at a price. Part of the price was the failure to subject abuses within the scientific perspective to an equally demanding critical analysis. These abuses do, in fact, exist. The proper level of analysis for such a critique is one dealing with science and social responsibility. Although the specifics of this analysis are largely unrelated to the purpose of this book, there are some general considerations which are relevant for finding solutions to the problems we have identified. Several of these considerations have been implied or referred to in passing, but they are sufficiently important that they need to be stated in their own right.

The blame for the abuses of the mental health movement must be placed on the scientific establishment as well as on the professional. The scientist, both individually and collectively through his associations, can no longer remain aloof from the world. He must walk and talk with the public. If he does not, the evolution of the social values necessary to harness science for the betterment of man will fail to occur, and all of mankind will be victimized. There are two very simple conceptual requirements, but ones that are difficult practically for science to fulfill. Both are necessary if the abuses of the mental health movement are to be resolved.

The first is the necessity to speak out about what is known and what is not known. For example, the scientific community sat back while a massive federal antidrug campaign advertised that LSD produced chromosome breakage, knowing all the time that the necessary data had not been collected and that caffeine and aspirin, among other readily available substances, produce breakage ten or more times as severe as that attributed to LSD. The credibility of science was damaged because it permitted a false claim to go unchallenged. Such silence was socially irresponsible, however, because current knowledge was abused for political reasons.

More recently, we have seen the abuse of psychiatry in Russia by the use of commitment as a means to suppress intellectual dissent, and the deliberate refusal of a world scientific congress on psychiatry to recognize that the issue even existed

203

despite appeals to its organizers.[4] The accomplice of silence is a failure to exercise the social responsibility of providing the public with information about what is and what is not consistent with current knowledge.

The silence is not hard to understand. Professional psychology has inflated scientific psychology to its current position of size and influence. Scientific psychology enjoys the economic resources and the power indirectly bestowed upon them by default. Likewise, to correct the misinformation in a drug abuse program could endanger federal funds for research in general or for the particular individuals or discipline involved. To acknowledge the Russian situation could disrupt the pursuit of personal ends at a world conference. Those who would speak out are silenced by their own colleagues who consistently and conspiratorially discredit the individual and claim such involvement as inappropriate.

The public posture of noninvolvement has been justified in terms of academic freedom and the necessity of science to remain above such issues. We must recognize that such a position is no longer viable. An informed public is necessary to articulate the collective social values needed to live in a scientific world. Further, it is important to maintain the credibility of science if we are to stop wholesale abuse of information for political purposes. Science must become part of the public sector. Scientific responsibility requires the public articulation of what science is doing and where it will lead if we are to have an open and free society which determines its own destiny. Otherwise, those who control science will determine the destiny of people; and what was to be the slave, giving all a better material life, will become the master.

The second requirement is for communication

with the public regarding the unfolding implications of science. In the case of the mental health movement, it means publicly dealing with the implications of behavior control. For example, what are the implications of permanently implanting in the brain electrodes which are capable of relieving anxiety, of electronically monitoring the psychophysiological response system at a central receiving station through miniature remote transmitters, and from this station triggering stimulation when needed? Can we envision this as a treatment program for patients? What about as a standard classroom procedure in public schools for monitoring attention, and activating, when necessary, central stimulation to raise attention and thus increase learning efficiency and help eliminate classroom behavior problems? The latter task is technically possible now and most certainly will be easy to engineer within the next decade or two at the very most. From a profession which brought us psychosurgery when it became technically possible, we can only expect implants as the next "benevolent" act of the mental health expert in behalf of public mental health.

Scientific responsibility requires widespread public dissemination of such information, because there is a need for public discussions and for public commissions. We must quickly get on with the debate regarding the implications of the behavioral and social sciences if we are to be the masters of our science. It is the debate—and the control which follows—which will ensure a free and open society. Such debate is necessary to allow science to fulfill values we will formulate, rather than to have the nonarticulated implications of science impose conditions we neither value nor choose.

Scientists react negatively to the word "control," for it implies loss of freedom. Not so. The capacity to select rationally the values around which our science will be framed is necessary to ensure a free and open society.

Thus, although the mental health movement poses a direct danger to a free and open society, and in many ways, is currently engaged in abuses, these are but immediate, temporary problems. A larger, more remote, long-term problem is the appropriate place of science and scientific responsibility in a modern society. If we are to solve the problem of the mental health ideology we need, as well, to move toward a more responsible role for science. The abuses of the mental health movement could not have proceeded without the silent, and irresponsible, accommodation provided, as when universities profit through expansion of the mental health market in ways which violate knowledge, or academic values, or both. Science must share in the blame as well as participate in the solution.

Commentary

It is perhaps not surprising that concepts of mental health, adjustment, and emotional maturity have become so firmly established. They may be seen as filling an ideological gap created by the age of materialism and relativism typical of twentieth-century American society. Their entrenchment, however, is no justification for their continued residency. Clinical psychology and psychiatry have filled this gap by providing a formula for life. Unfortunately, the biological and social sciences cannot provide ideological answers. To act as if they could is to obscure the prospect for the future. The time to come to grips with how to live with the knowledge being provided by the biological and social sciences is now. The new information will open doors of possibility that did not exist before, but which ultimately must rest on human values. Clinical psychology and psychiatry came of age at a time when a market existed and they fulfilled a temporary need. But to continue to cling to the mental health expert is to perpetuate the delay in coping with our contemporary problems of living—including madness.

My purpose is not so much to crusade for what I feel is correct, as it is to raise issues which must be dealt with. It is all arbitrary, but the way the various issues are seen is no small matter. We are touching on matters of considerable social importance.

One might question whether this book has presented an overidealized view of science. I think not. Once psychiatry, clinical psychology and their collective public image can get on with the business of applying verifiable information and of opening new avenues for dealing with human behavior, solutions to problems of deeply felt humanistic concern will follow. I expect to see this within my lifetime.

The view is simple. Human behavior, be it pants wetting, obsessive symptoms, schizophrenia, or tenderness and love, is what people do and say and feel. These are behaviors that individuals show in various situations. *It is their behavior that they must be held responsible for,* and it is their behavior that we will come to have greater and greater control over. It is rapidly becoming an urgent necessity to take current scientific perspectives and turn them into a workable prospect for the future.

notes

Chapter 1. Introduction

1. The material from *Malleus Maleficarum* was taken from a translation by Reverend Montague Summers of a manuscript copy dated 1489. The translation was published in a limited edition by John Rodker, publisher, Great Britain, in 1928. The copy used here is in the rare book collection of the University of Illinois library. The passages cited are from pages 120, 103, 117, 149, and 225 respectively, of that book.

2. Quoted in A. Deutsch, *The Mentally Ill in America* (New York: Columbia University Press, 1949), p. 80.

3. More detailed accounts of various physical treatments can be found in any reliable psychiatric

textbook, such as the one by A.P. Noyes and L.C. Kolb, *Modern Clinical Psychiatry*, 6th edition, published by W.B. Sanders. Since Dr. Noyes' death in 1963, this classic psychiatric book was continued under the authorship of Dr. Kolb with the 8th edition appearing in 1973.

4. The first quote is from *Malleus Maleficarum* (see note 1) and the second from *Modern Clinical Psychiatry* (see note 3).

Chapter 2. A brief historical perspective

1. E. Kraeplin, *Clinical Psychiatry*, translated from the German by A. Ross Diefendorf and published in the United States by Macmillan, 1907.

2. An excellent medical history of the period is G. Zilboorg and G.W. Henry, *A History of Medical Psychology* (New York: Norton, 1941).

3. The picture may be found on page 49 of A. Deutsch, *The Shame of the States* (New York: Harcourt Brace, 1948).

4. See D. Peterson, *The Clinical Study of Social Behavior* (New York: Appleton-Century-Crofts, 1968) for a further comparison and discussion of the issues surrounding treatment in state hospitals and the alternatives available.

5. Joint Commission on Mental Illness and Health, *Action for Mental Health* (New York: Basic Books, 1961).

Chapter 3. Normality-abnormality: by what criterion

1. W. Scott, "Research definitions of mental health and illness," *Psychological Bulletin,* 1958, 55, 29-45.

Chapter 5. The diagnostic system

1. *Diagnostic and Statistical Manual of Mental Disorders* was published in its basic form by the American Psychiatric Association in 1952. The manual, however, is continually updated. The most

recent vote by the membership in 1974 removed homosexuality from the list of mental disorders.

2. R.W. Payne, "Cognitive abnormalities," in H.J. Eysenck (Ed.), *Handbook of Abnormal Psychology* (New York: Basic Books, 1961).

3. L. Irwin and K.E. Renner, "The effects of praise and censure on the performance of schizophrenics," *Journal of Abnormal Psychology,* 1969, 74, 221-226.

4. L.C. Robbins, "The accuracy of parental recall of aspects of child development and child rearing practices," *Journal of Abnormal and Social Psychology,* 1963, 66, 261-270.

5. A. Buss, *Psychopathology* (New York: Wiley, 1966), chapters 12, 13, and 14.

Chapter 6. Mental illness versus behavior disorder

1. T. Szasz, *The Myth of Mental Illness* (New York: Hoeber-Harper, 1961). And, "What psychiatry can and cannot do," *Harpers,* February, 1964.

2. For a detailed discussion of this issue by a lawyer with respect to mental illness and a variety of other problem behaviors (e.g., alcoholism, drug use, delinquency, poverty), see N.B. Kittrie, *The Right to Be Different* (Baltimore: Johns Hopkins Press, 1971). He discusses a variety of treatments that may be imposed on persons against their will, such as sterilization after having illegitimate babies, although the principal focus is on sanctions that are justified on the grounds of mental illness.

3. H.A. Davidson, "The commitment procedures and their legal implications," in S. Arieti (Ed.), *American Handbook of Psychiatry,* Vol. 2 (New York: Basic Books, 1959), page 1902.

4. T. Szasz, *Law, Liberty and Psychiatry* (New York: Macmillan, 1963), especially page 63. See also note 2.

5. E.S. Sulzer, "Demagogues and mental health:

A look at both sides," *Community Mental Health Journal*, 1965, 1, 14-18.

6. See notes 1 and 4.

Chapter 7. A pair of alternatives

1. W. McCord and J. McCord, *The Psychopath: An Essay on the Criminal Mind* (New York: Van Nostrand, 1964).

2. B. Bettelheim, *Dialogues With Mothers* (New York: Macmillan, 1962), chapter 2.

3. C.H. Madsen, "Positive reinforcement in the toilet training of a normal child: A case report," in L.P. Ullman and L. Krasner (Eds.), *Case Studies in Behavioral Modification* (New York: Holt, Rinehart and Winston, 1965).

4. D. Blain, "Everyone should have a periodic checkup for our no. 1 health problem: Mental illness," *Philadelphia Bulletin*, Sunday Magazine, October, 18, 1964.

Chapter 9. Clinical decisions

1. H.G. Gough, E. Wenk, and V.V. Rozynko, "Parole outcome as predicted from the CPI, the MMPI, and a base expectancy table," *Journal of Consulting Psychology*, 1965, 70, 531-541.

2. Paul Meehl's classic and often cited work is *Clinical Versus Statistical Prediction* (Minneapolis: University of Minnesota Press, 1954). The twenty years of research subsequent to the publication of his book have only served to reaffirm its basic conclusions.

3. J. Masling, "The influence of situational and interpersonal variables in projective testing," *Psychological Bulletin*, 1960, 57, 65-85.

4. A.R. Jensen, "Personality," *Annual Review of Psychology*, 1958, 9.

5. W. Mischel, *Personality Assessment* (New York: Wiley, 1968).

Chapter 10. Psychotherapy

1. Freud published many case studies to illustrate and to document the usefulness of his techniques. The reference in the text is to J. Breuer and S. Freud, *Studies in Hysteria*, translated by A.A. Brill and published in 1936 by the Nervous and Mental Disease Publishing Co. The reference to caramel candy is to the case study by Charles Madsen on toilet training which was described in Chapter 7; that particular case, however, is but one example from a larger collection edited by L.P. Ullman and L. Krasner, *Case Studies in Behavior Modification* (New York: Holt, Rinehart and Winston, 1965).

2. P. Meehl, "Psychotherapy," *Annual Review of Psychology,* 1955, 6.

3. H.J. Eysenck, "The effects of psychotherapy: An evaluation," *Journal of Consulting Psychology,* 1952, 16, 319-324. And, "The effects of psychotherapy," in H.J. Eysenck (Ed.), *Handbook of Abnormal Psychology* (New York: Basic Books, 1961). Eysenck's basic findings in 1974 still remain unchallenged.

4. J. Wolpe, *Psychotherapy by Reciprocal Inhibition* (Palo Alto, Calif.: Stanford University Press, 1958).

Chapter 11. An overview

1. See *Saturday Review*, March 26, 1966; *Life*, March 4, 1966; *Ladies' Home Journal*, May 1966; or H. Painter, *Mark, I Love You* (New York: Simon and Schuster, 1967).

2. C.H. Thigpen and H.M. Cleckley, "Some reflections on psychoanalysis, hypnosis, and faith healing," in J. Wolpe, A. Salter, and L.J. Reyna (Eds.), *The Conditioning Therapies* (New York: Holt, Rinehart and Winston, 1964).

Chapter 12. Community psychology

1. Z. Medvedev and R. Medvedev, *A Question of Madness* (New York: Macmillan, 1971).

2. R. Reiff, "Mental health manpower and institutional change," in E.L. Cowen, E.A. Gardner, and M. Zax (Eds.), *Emergent Approaches to Mental Health Problems* (New York: Appleton-Century-Crofts, 1967).

3. C.W. Thomas, "Psychologists, psychology, and the black community," in C. Spielberger (Ed.), *Current Topics in Clinical and Community Psychology*, Volume 3 (New York: Academic Press, 1971).

4. V.L. Allen (Ed.), *Psychological Factors in Poverty* (Chicago: Markham, 1970).

5. M.B. Smith and N. Hobbs, "The community and the community mental health center," *American Psychologist*, 1966, 21, 499-509.

Chapter 13. Action for mental health

1. W. Schofield, *Psychotherapy: The Purchase of Friendship* (Englewood Cliffs, N.J.: Prentice-Hall, 1964).

2. A. Mariner, "A critical look at professional education in the mental health field," *American Psychologist*, 1967, 22, 271-281.

3. J. Bockoven, *Moral Treatment in American Psychiatry* (New York: Springer, 1963).

4. I.F. Stone, "Betrayal by Psychiatry," *New York Review of Books*, February 10, 1972, pp. 7-14. See also Chapter 12, note 1.

name index

subject index

217

About the Author
K. Edward Renner, Ph.D.

The author is a professor in the Department of Psychology at the University of Illinois at Urbana. His previous affiliation was with the University of Pennsylvania, where he served as an assistant professor.

In addition to his work on numerous committees at Illinois, Dr. Renner reviews manuscripts for a half-dozen professional journals; he is also engaged in psychological research.

Dr. Renner has written articles for many journals, including *Journal of Individual Psychology, Journal of Applied Psychology, American Psychologist, Journal of Comparative and Physiological Psychology, Journal of Experimental Psychology, Journal of Abnormal Psychology,* and *Psychological Reports.*

He earned his B.S. degree at Pennsylvania State University, and his M.A. and Ph.D degrees at Northwestern University. He has won over a dozen awards, scholarships, appointments, and grants.